Galloping
Catastrophe

MUSINGS OF A MENOPAUSAL WOMAN

JENNIFER KENNEDY

ISBN: 978-1-09-674251-7

Illustrations: Daniel McCloskey

Cover design & typesetting:
David Siddall Multimedia, Monmouth, UK
www.davidsiddall.com

Dedications

This book is dedicated to a number of wonderful
Galloping Catastrophes in my life:

Gill and Judith – for the way you live your life your way and inspire
me to do the same. And for the drunken rambling nights of course...

Kathleen – for being the kindest most supportive wonderful
human being on this earth and for (eventually) forgiving me

Fiona S, Rosie and Mary – who have known me half a century
and know my light and my darkness – and always focus on the light.

Jen F – for being so utterly amazing during some of the worst
months of my life – you'll never know how much it meant.

Arlene – you're not quite a Galloping Catastrophe yet – I've known
you since I babysat you as a tiny wee toddler and never cease to be
amazed at the totally amazing woman you have become. You are, and
always will be, the little sister I never had.

Helen, Fiona M, Bev, Tracey, Gillybean Ann G, Little Cuz Jane,
Chellbelle, Auntie Mary and everyone else who supported me writing
my blog and my book.

And to all the Galloping Catastrophes of my blog who encouraged
me to write this book.

And also for Sweet Dog.

So happy that you are all in my life!

Contents

Introduction

If you are reading this – the chances are you are menopausal/ peri-menopausal or know someone who is.

If you are menopausal, you probably got up today after a crap night's sleep where possibly you had to change your nightwear as it was saturated in sweat. You probably started your day plucking hairs from your chin cursing the irony that the hair on your head is starting to thin. Getting dressed was probably a nightmare as you sought to disguise the menopausal middle. You may have planned to have muesli for breakfast but in the end, had a roll and sausage and maybe a cake. By 11am it's likely you will have wanted to tell various people to 'go to fuck' and when they get there to just keep fucking off 'til they have fucked right off! Indeed you may have given in to those desires and possibly and have now lost a job/ partner/friend as a result. At 3pm it's likely you would have been hit with a ten-ton wrecking ball otherwise known as mid-afternoon menopausal exhaustion...

Sound familiar?

If you are reading this because you know a menopausal woman. In that case, you probably are wondering what the actual fuck has happened to this person – has an alien taken over her body and mind? Perhaps you tiptoe around her due to the volcanic eruption that takes place if you so much as breathe too loudly. Maybe you are concerned about her finances as you keep finding her in tears watching day time telly using her credit card to try and 'Save the Donkey'.

Sound familiar?

There is of course an outside chance you are not quite there yet and want to know what might be coming your way – if so, my advice is to close the book now and enjoy blissful ignorance then return to it when you get the notion to stab people and start forgetting things like your children's names and the route into work.

This book is to share my experiences of the menopause and have you realise it's not just you. It features my lovely Sweet Dog – who is the bestest menopausal support there is! It's not a '12 step programme' to 'fix you'. Nor is it a happy-clappy guide trying to persuade you that daily spoon of hemp oil and regular kale smoothies will magically transform you. It won't help you find your 'inner self'. These were the only books I could find when I tried to find help. One showed a woman being given a piggyback by her husband as he ran through a field – both laughing in joy. Seriously? If I tried that I'd break my partners back! Another showed a woman full of health and vitality striding through the countryside and recommended supplements that would probably cost £100s per month. I had spent most of that day in pyjamas (the menopausal woman's outfit of choice) watching Loose Women on catch-up while eating cheap chocolate and trying to work out how I'd get to payday without going overdrawn. I've read articles from women claiming it is wonderful to be 50+ as they are financially secure, their mortgages are paid off and they have a good pension to look forward to. Well, I beg to feckin differ! No that's not me – mortgaged up to the hilt, skint, no pension to speak of and looking forward to an old age working in B&Q or for SAGA. No point in buying this book if you are looking for a role model or an inspirational story of finding joy in the menopausal years.

In 1966, Doctor Robert Wilson referred to menopausal women as '*Galloping Catastrophes*'. It was meant in a derogatory way. But I didn't take it like that – it sums me up exactly. So I have reclaimed it. This book is for all the other '*Galloping Catastrophes*' out there. It talks through my experiences of the menopause so far. And while Kale smoothies and Hemp Oil and Big Walks can help – we all know that reading about others disastrous experience and laughing/crying 'til the tears run down your legs is the best 'self-help' there is

It isn't intended to be read all the way through from start to finish – although you can if you want (I would never mess with a decision a menopausal woman made). It is more of a dip in and dip out. Had a fucker of a day – read about mine. Can't fit into your clothes – read about my experiences. And feel just that wee bit better that it's not just you!

So for *Galloping Catastrophes* everywhere – this one's for you!

CHAPTER 1

Fat class for the fat lass

In this chapter, I bring to you – my meno-musings on the ongoing battle with the Menopausal Midriff!

I am 4 stone heavier than I was when all this menopause malarkey started. And most of it is on my tummy which I think may soon be eligible for a postcode all to itself. I slipped in the shower the other day and my first thought wasn't about possible concussion – it was, 'Oh God they are going to find me naked'.

What can you do? Well, I tried to help myself – I decided to join a 'Fat Class'. There is a plethora so I just chose the nearest one to my flat as didn't want to walk too far

I have been to a Fat Class before – I swore I would never return after the first meeting was spent listening to someone called Big Mags crying her eyes out as she had 'stuck to the plan completely apart from 2 Jaffa Cakes when she was watching Coronation Street on Wednesday' and still managed to gain 4lbs which has pushed her back over 20 stones. I suspected she was lying. And I suspected the leader knew she was lying but we all colluded to make her believe it was maybe just a wee gland issue or something. The next week I had to endure some skinny kid waffling on about how she couldn't believe she had lost 3lbs after she had got drunk all weekend, had 2 kebabs and a Chinese takeaway. It was my first week and I had stuck to the 'formula' all week and lost one pound. ONE POUND!! And I was starving and mad so stopped for a fish supper, a black forest gateau and a bottle of wine on the way home and that was the end of that!

But I am desperate and I cannot bear another summer of the dreaded chub-rub under my summer dresses. My button popped off my biggest trousers at work and I was mortified (though I sewed it back on an inch closer to the buttonhole so every cloud and all that). And I am so over shopping in Evans! And people keep telling me you can stuff your face on the 'Fat Class for the Fat Lass' plan and still lose weight. So it seemed to suit me to the ground.

So off I went – after one last splurge on takeaway, wine, crisps and a huge bag of Cadbury's chocolate eclairs. Sort of like a last hoorah before joining the slimming mafia.

And God it was boring. The big long talk for newbies on Choices/Fat Foods/Naughty Foods/Super-Healthy foods that none of us really listened to as we were desperately trying to find the page that told us how much chocolate, cake and wine we could have in a day.

Then everyone individually said what had led them to gain or lose weight the previous week. There wasn't much variation on the theme of eating too much/eating what you were supposed to. A huge round of applause followed each person and my head was really hurting because of the wine. I had a stone in my shoe and it was annoying me but I kept pressing down on it enjoying the release from the boredom the pain gave me.

A discussion of how we could all do better next week then ensued. One of the older ladies shared her tip of getting her husband to hide her false teeth at 5 pm so she couldn't eat anything else that night. I almost spat out my 'Fat Lass' bar (a product that costs a fortune but apparently will curb your chocolate cravings. This turned out to be a lie – but more on that later) laughing. But I was the only one – everyone else was nodding earnestly. I swear a couple were thinking of having their teeth removed so they could do the same.

Then it was the dreaded weigh in. Another newbie was just before me and dressed in heavy jeans and a heavy sweater. She was dripping with sweat and I thought aha a fellow hot flusher! But no... she told me that she also had two t-shirts under the jumper because wearing really heavy clothes the first week then lighter ones the next week means you lose much more weight that week. Well I beg to feckin differ – but I kept quiet... each to their own

I had to set a target weight – I was going to go for my weight before this menopausal madness all started. That means a loss of around 40lb. That seemed like an awful lot so I decide to keep 10lbs as a kind of souvenir of the menopause so that brings it down to 30 which seems a bit more manageable.

Finally my turn for the weight in. Oh, God. I pull my trainers off and get on the scales – that bloody stone is now stuck to my sock. I reach down to brush it away. But it isn't a stone. It is a Cadbury's chocolate eclair! The weigher in person looks at me in what I can only say is disgust as I peel it off my sock. I can't see a bin and my diet hasn't officially started yet and I am quite stressed – so I just pop it into my mouth. I don't know why I did that really – just a reflex action to a sweetie I suspect. But it is an embarrassment I can ponder when menopausal insomnia strikes at 3am as I have to spend now being totally mortified at the figure on the scale. Then totally shocked that the woman doesn't say 'oh you don't seem that big' and just calmly writes the colossal figure down. Surely she can see that I must have heavy bones and make some kind of comment. But nope. Sometimes I wonder if I have reverse body dysmorphia – I can look at my body and think 'oh not too bad' 'til the number flashes up in neon lights on the scales as indisputable evidence.

Hey ho – off I went with the books and a determination to get thin. I had so many tips from the leader – it all seemed too good to be true. Because it was!! I have listed some of the Fat Lass tips I received on losing weight and compared them to the cold reality:

Fat Lass Tip:

Lovely 'Fat Lass' bars – great when you crave a bit of chocolate – just have one and your cravings will be gone. The leader actually said they were 'the answer to her prayers'. Though she maybe just meant the amount of commission she got on them – they are not cheap!

Reality:

I can talk with great authority on this as I ate the entire boxful on the first night. They do not take away your cravings – they taste weird. And make your tummy cramp if you eat too many. I am going back to Galaxy's. (just as an aside if my prayers were answered they would not in any way involve a box of Fat Lass bars – so God if you are listening – a nice car, house by the sea, and most importantly to be able to fit my arse into a pair of size 14 jeans. World peace and all the rest too would be good – but whatever – don't forget about the jeans thing)

Fat Lass Tip:

Put grapes in the freezer and when you take them out they taste like boiled sweeties.

Reality:

No they don't – they taste like frozen grapes!

Fat Lass Tip:

You can go to the chippie with the family so you won't feel left out.

Reality:

Yes – but when you read the small print you can have a fish supper but with no chips and only if you peel all the batter off! And have a tomato salad with it. Aye right!!! Coz peeling batter off your fish and not having any chips while everyone else gets tucked into their beer battered fish and huge portions of fries really makes you feel part of it!

3

Fat Lass Tip:

Chop up a butternut squash, spray with 'fry light' and stick in the oven for 20 mins – they come out just like chips from the chippie.

Reality:

A butternut squash is not squashy and has the texture of a rock rather than butter! Trying to chop it will bring on a menopausal rage of immense proportions. Once you have spent 20 mins peeling trying to chop and scooping out the seeds you won't give a feck what it tastes like. Which is just as well – coz they are nothing like chippie chips. They taste of a rock hard vegetable – coz that is what they are!

Fat Lass Tip:

If you crave crisps, just sprinkle salt on some kale, blast with some spray oil and put in the oven.

Reality:

Again I beg to feckin differ – nothing like a packet of Walkers Cheese and Onion. Nothing at all.

Fat Lass Tip:

Choose wisely and you can enjoy a full fry-up in the morning.

Reality:

Yep – but you have to have the special 'Fat Lass' sausages which are so awful even my Sweet Dog would not eat them (and she has been known to eat her own vomit which gives you an idea of her standards), no fat on your bacon, no potato scones, no toast covered with butter, no square sausage – basically nothing that makes a fry up a fry-up!

Fat Lass Tip:

Slice bananas and freeze them – then you can mash them up and it is like lovely banana ice cream.

Reality:

You will forget about them until your partner discovers them in the freezer 4 weeks later and screams thinking they are frozen fingers then says 'what the actual fuck' several times when you try to explain.

Fat Lass Tip:

You don't need real Ferrero Rocher – just mix a Ryveta with a tiny bit of Nutella and a little syrup and put it in the fridge – tastes the exact same.

Reality:

This is a big lie – but TBH I didn't really fall for it – if perhaps you could have a jar of Nutella with maybe a Ryveta to dip in it that might be different.

I could go on – but basically, in order to have a weight loss next week, I have to eat more healthy food, less unhealthy food and take more exercise. Sweet Dog is most happy with the 'more exercise' bit so at least someone is happy...

And perhaps wear lighter clothes...

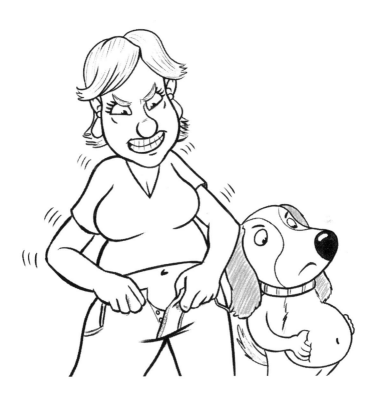

CHAPTER 2

Becoming invisible

In this chapter, I bring to you – my meno-musings on my Menopausal Superpower.

You too may have discovered that when you hit menopausal age you too discover a permanent cloak of invisibility.

I have definitely become the Invisible Woman (except to my Sweet Dog who adores me and 'sees' me all the time especially when I say 'walkies'). Which is ironic given I am bigger than I have ever been in my life.

And this isn't just me being maudlin. A recent poll found that 46 was the average age that women start to feel invisible.

Take a recent trip into work. I am waiting to get on the tram and a man steps practically through me and stands one inch in front of me so he can get on first. He didn't see me at all as he rushed for the last available seat. He didn't quite knock me over as I am a bit like a weeble in that I wobble a lot – but I don't fall down. He didn't seem me in fact 'til I 'accidentally' stood on his foot. At the next stop though he leapt off the seat as if there was firework about to go off up his arse so he could help a gorgeous 20 something woman off the tram with her bag. I nicked his seat quick smart. He saw me then!

At the lift at work, two people just pushed straight past me, not even interrupting their conversation to acknowledge me. They didn't ask what floor I want to get out at and just hit Floor 9 for themselves. They notice me though when I pressed all the buttons from Floor 1 to Floor 9 then departed on Floor one happy in the knowledge it will jolt up one floor at a time. I probably should not admit this but I also let out a fart of the silent but deadly type (I had a tandoori the night before). Ha. (I was going to take the stairs every time I was only doing one floor but I am going to wait 'til I get a Fitbit so that I can officially record it each time).

I go to the shops for some chocolate and a guy comes in and shouts over my head for fags – '20 of my usual fags mate'. The shopkeeper also can't see me as he goes to serve him first. But they see me when I say 'EXCUSE ME I think you'll find I was here first' because invisible women aren't supposed to speak up for themselves – they are supposed to accept their lot. Well, I beg to feckin differ! Not me. Not now. Not ever. I'd recommend it – speaking up for yourself becomes easier and easier the more you do it.

The snotty woman who told me haughtily not to take two of the (postage stamp sized) towels when I made my yearly visit to the gym that I pay £60 a month to not use – I told her 'I beg to feckin differ – I am taking them and get the manager ready for me when I came out to discuss further if it is a problem'.

The shop assistant who gazed above my head while holding her hand out for my money – she finally saw me after I just stood still refusing to be ignored – and finally asked me for the money and even said please.

The guy who marched past me when I stood aside for him who turned in shock when I shouted 'you're welcome'.

The young woman who pushed up against me on the sale rail and looked at me in shock when I said 'I think the phrase you are looking for is 'excuse me'. She was so stunned that I had a moment of horror thinking she was maybe deaf and mute and I had just been disabilityist – but turns out she was just totally shocked about an invisible woman actually talking.

My friend's 17 year-old who said that one of the 'celebs' on her magazine was a feminist because she earned lots of money and did what she wanted with her body – who had the good grace to look embarrassed when she realised I wasn't invisible as I fell about laughing explaining to her that getting your arse and tits out is fine if you want to but for God's sake don't call it feminism.

I mean I know I'm not exactly Rosa Parks – but there is a thrill in small moments of being very visible – and giving zero fucks about what anyone thinks about it.

The list goes on. Doors swing back in my face. Bar people ignore me as the young and the beautiful walk in front of me to be served first. I am only represented in incontinence and nutritional supplement adverts – I don't exist to the sexy car adverts. Nobody stands up for me on the bus. Hairdressers gaze at themselves in the mirror as they work on my hair. Construction workers don't lift their eyes from their doughnut and newspaper when I pass. On one memorable occasion, I spent £200 on having my hair darkened and cut and felt most self-conscious the next day 'til I realised not one fecker had noticed. Sweet Dog is a blessing – always thrilled to see me – once noticing me even when I was a good mile away and charging towards me full of joy.

I can't decide if this invisibility is a good or a bad thing. I sit in Coffee Shops with a book and a Latte without having to endure some fool 'talking' to me about what I am reading/why I am there etc. I can go out and no-one yells 'cor look at the arse on that'. No more unwanted attention. Because I am an invisible woman. And often, I am grateful for the silence.

How much further can I can take it? Would I be invisible to the John Lewis security guard? I ponder as I finger their lovely but very expensive silk scarves. I resist though. I am waiting 'til I am in my 70s before I start properly shoplifting. If I don't get caught I will sell my gains for cash to buy butter and chocolate and big purple hats. If I do get caught, prison is likely to be an improvement on the only care homes I will be able to afford (because the government took all my money away and won't give it back as a pension 'til I am 107 which was NOT the deal I signed up to). Three good meals a day, lots of company; my own room with telly; access to education etc. My mum is a little concerned about this retirement plan and thinks I should up the pension contributions but I beg to feckin differ.

I was talking to a head teacher friend of mine, Michelle, about this last week – and she was feeling rather pleased with herself. She had discovered an on-line poll her pupils had put together – rating her and the other female teachers out of 20. While having to be outwardly disapproving of the poll which objectified women – she was pleasantly surprised to find she had scored 19 as many of her younger and, as she perceived, more attractive colleagues had scored much lower. She put it down to her healthy vegetarian lifestyle and regular exercise plan with occasional shots of Botox.

However... her joy was deflated the next day when it was uncovered that the score was the number of pints of beer the boys who had created the poll felt they would have to drink before 'shagging' the teacher in question.

When she told me about it we both laughed so much we wee-d a bit. And we realised that if she had been given that score at the age of 25 she would have been devastated. But with invisibility comes a subtler and stronger power than sexuality. An ability to laugh at yourself. An ability to speak up and be heard because you don't really care any more about what people think.

Try it – it's addictive... All hail the Invisible Woman!

CHAPTER 3

Menopausal Hypochondria

In this chapter, I bring to you – my meno-musings on my hypochondria.

In the year running up to my menopausal diagnosis, I had been at the doctor's so often that I actually dropped a Christmas card in for the receptionists (my surgery's receptionists are lovely unlike the stereotypical dragons you often hear about). The doctors are lovely too – showing great patience as I regularly popped in convinced I had one or a combination of:

- *Alzheimer's* (as can't remember anything)
- *Early-onset Dementia* (as above)
- *Underactive Thyroid* (gained 20lbs in a year)
- *Diabetes* (craving sugar)
- *Vitamin D deficiency* (muscles feel weak and am just so tired all the time)
- *Depression* (just want to lie in bed all the time, lost my 'zest for life', cry a lot)
- *Bipolar Syndrome* (am manically high which leads to many purchases of shoes and handbags then so low which leads to lots of rum and chocolate)
- *Ovarian Cancer* (my belly is so swollen I look 6 months pregnant)
- *Borderline Personality Disorder* (I love myself then I hate myself).

It was a locum. Dr Nightingale (that was her real name... how cool!) that finally suggested I may be menopausal. I was highly offended. 'Very much MENSTRUAL, thank you very much! Every 26 days without fail' I told her while I desperately tried to work out when the last period was. 'Test me' I demanded – there is so much of my blood floating around in laboratories after all the other tests I thought why not. No point she said – tests are inconclusive. But if there was a test – I am pretty sure it would show positive for peri-menopause. Positive! Nothing bloody positive about that I thought. Perimenopause – the worst of both worlds. Still having periods but menopausal at the same time. She did a battery of other tests to reassure me that it wasn't anything else. Then she finished by reassuring me this was all perfectly normal – a bit like a practice for the real thing which I found less than helpful. Like PMT on crack is a better description

Menopause. Yes of course I had heard of it – and I knew I would probably have to go through it at some point. Joan Stopes from Finance at work went through it last year, she called it 'the change' and bored the arse of anyone who shows even a vague interest – when she wasn't having days on the sick. She used to sweat profusely, regularly pull a fan from her drawer and whizz it dramatically in front of her four or five times a day. She then went off long term sick after telling the HR Advisor to 'shove your absence policy up your arse' and we got an email from HR saying the company was being supportive to Joan and reminding us it was an 'attendance policy' not an absence policy and we should all remember to use that term . But she was old – with grey frizzy hair. And elasticated beige trousers. So although I knew at some point I would go through it – it seemed a very long way into the future.

When I did think about it – which was rare – I suppose I felt I would be a bit more 'Helen Mirren' about the whole thing. Elegant and Slim. Floating my way through it gently like a summer breeze. I certainly wouldn't be like Joan.

Three days after my visit to the surgery I got a call telling me to come into the surgery. Oh no... OH NO... What is wrong with me? There must be something. I go into meltdown and try to call the surgery back but it is closed. I try desperately what all the blood tests were for but I have forgotten them all. I call my nurse friend in panic (poor Vanessa Sendler – she now shows as one of my favourite numbers).

'Did they ask you to bring someone with you?' she asks sounding a little exasperated. 'No' I reply. 'Well it probably isn't that bad' she reassures me.

But I am terrified now – I knew I was really ill and it wasn't the menopause!! Told you so told you so told you so.... On the way in I try to decide what to do when they ask if I want palliative care – do I want to endure treatment for a few extra months. I don't want Sweet Dog to see my ill. I cuddle her close trying not to cry – who will look after my lovely Sweet Dog when I am gone. You don't ever expect that your dog will have to bury you. I call my partner to discuss but they tell me I am being a drama queen and so far there is nothing wrong with me. They will bloody regret it when I am given my diagnosis!!!

Well, there was something wrong this time – an Underactive Thyroid. I almost leap out my chair and punch the air. The Doctor tells me it is common in menopausal women and asks me if I know what it means. I am so excited... 'It's why I am fat and knackered' I explain 'and you just give me tablets and I will be thin and energetic again'. I have learned all I know from Doctor Google I say proudly. Doctor Nightingale says that I am being a bit over simplistic and not 100 per cent accurate and proceeds to give a more medical description because she needs to prove that she has done 7 years at medical school. She also tries to talk about HRT and its benefits but of course, I know I am not menopausal so I barely listen as I imagine joining the world of the thin and wide awake club!

I bounce out of the surgery clutching my prescription with the GP no doubt writing 'possible bipolar' on my notes.

CHAPTER 4

Appointment at the Menopause Clinic

In this chapter, I bring to you – my meno-musings on my recent trip to the Menopause Clinic.

I had to pretty much stage a menopausal coup at the GP's surgery to get this referral. I had returned after getting a diagnosis of underactive thyroid and thinking that the tablets would cure all. They didn't. A friend told me about the menopausal clinic and I was determined to get an appointment. The coup was successful due to my relatively recently developed skill of complete obstinate stubbornness. I pretty much told Doctor Nightingale I wasn't leaving the surgery 'til I had it. No, I didn't want anti-depressants. No, I didn't want to take HRT 'and see how it went'. NO, NO, NO, I want to talk to a specialist who has more than 5 minutes to talk to me and actually knows a bit about what I am going through. I was about to add 'and isn't bloody ten years old' but felt that might be ageist and you have to be careful about being 'ist' these days.

I am lucky to live in Edinburgh so at least I have a Menopause Clinic to be referred to even though getting an audience with the queen may well be easier than getting an appointment there.

So it took six months from then to actually getting the momentous appointment. I decided to get up early and walk. I am determined to get my 10,000 steps a day in. So 40 minutes later I am almost at Chambers Street with 10 mins to spare. But I can't bloody find it. I check... OFFS – it isn't Chambers Street it is Chalmers Street. Chalmers Street – WTF – I check my Google Maps and find it – thank God for technology. I have forgotten my earphones so will just have to play the directions out loud and if people don't like it they can feck off – it will make up for the number of times I have had to listen to crap coming out of other people's mobiles.

'STARTING ROUTE TO... CHALMERS SEXUAL HEALTH CENTRE' Oh no – where is the volume? – I forgot I had put it up when I was listening to Spotify this morning and dancing like no-one was watching. A bunch of workmen smirk but say nothing. It is Edinburgh after all. If it was Glasgow I feel the response may have been rather more raucous.

I am sure this isn't the right way and am starting to get irritable. Very irritable. Stupid Google Maps is only showing driving instructions despite me hitting the walking person symbol several times. I have had a hot flush and am soaked. I am knackered and my foot is hurting from all the walking. And I am going to be late. And I don't want to have to wait another six months for another appointment.

My phone rings – well 'Facetimes'. My niece Fiona Pankhurst downloaded it for me as I am clueless and here she is – brill she knows Edinburgh like the back of her hand. 'Hi Honey' I say – waiting for her cheery response.

"I AM LOOKING AT YOUR EAR AGAIN!' she shouts.

I keep forgetting that with Facetime you don't put your phone to your ear. I swing it back round.

I remember taking the piss out my mum when she got her first computer and carefully printed a letter out then Tippexed over the mistakes. I suspect the younger generation now look at me in a similar way.

Anyway, she hasn't a clue where Chalmers Street and although that means I am still lost – I am very glad she doesn't know where it is. She hangs up when I ask if she saw any wax in my ear – I worry a bit about this as my hair is up a lot just now due to the heat and hot flushes.

I see a taxi – thank God – and flag it down. 'Where to Love?' the driver says.

Oh No – I can't say the Sexual Health Centre. I can't. So I say "Chalmers Street please – number 2".

But he is not deterred. 'Is that the Dental Clinic love' he says. Oh God this is soohhh embarrassing. I decide I will try and come across as a Doctor – that will work – I am a Doctor with a very important job at the Sexual Health Clinic. I say confidently 'actually I'm off to Sexual Health Clinic'. Then I start worrying about something my partner said the other day – 'if there was a gift I could give you it would be a higher self-esteem'. I said that I beg to feckin differ – I'd prefer a bottle of Chanel Number 5 or some of that lovely blue Clarins hydrating moisturiser. My birthday was coming up and experience has taught me to be directive about gifts. I thought my self-esteem was OK but here I am trying to be a Doctor because I am worried the taxi driver will think I have VD so maybe they had a point.

My phone pipes up interrupting my musings. "Turn RIGHT for Chalmers Sexual Health Centre". The taxi driver glares at me in his rear view mirror – 'are you checking the route hen?'. I notice I am no longer a 'love'.

'Sorry, sorry – stupid phone'' I say and wonder about doing a pretend call to a pretend secretary about pretend patients. Then I remember I am nearly fifty and then I worry that perhaps I have Walter Mitty syndrome.

Finally get there. Why is the bloody Menopause Clinic part of a Sexual Health Centre? WHY? WHY? It's like a sick joke – haha menopausal women who are likely to be feeling fat, ugly and with no desire in sex whatsoever – come into our sexual health clinic. I am a little jealous of the young who are waiting – because at that age I wouldn't have needed a sexual health clinic as... well basically I wasn't having sex. I regret that now – if I had my time again I would shag whenever the desire took me and wear my grass stains with pride. Feck my body was smoking then and my libido was high. Why didn't I just give myself up to the moment? And have lots of moments one after the other. Instead of 'waiting'. And after all that waiting ending up with a fucktard with zero Emotional Intelligence. Nah – get out and sow the wild oats is my advice (unless you are my niece in which case hang on 'til at least the age of 35)

And finally I am seen. I see Doctor Alexis Lennox and see this as a sign. I love the name Alexis and often when I get my coffee I lie and tell the Barista that is my name so they scribble it on the cup and for a few minutes I am Alexis – strong and powerful yet sophisticated. She is so lovely and kind that I start to cry. This is a new menopausal symptom – I am much more familiar with the mood swings the temper and the irritability.

She is patient and gives me tissues. She is slightly thrown when I tell her about using her name in the coffee house but very collected apart from that. I can see myself in the mirror behind the Doctor and it's not pretty. I wish cried like Sinead O'Connor in that video – solitary tears dropping gracefully one by one. I just look like a weeping blotchy burst couch. And my hair has gone all funny.

Anyway, we have a lovely chat in the end. Well, she talks mainly and I sob and hiccough a lot. I do think if they gave a cup of tea and maybe a couple of Jaffa Cakes the experience would be much more enjoyable. I suggest this but she just smiles as if I made a joke. She shows me the leaflet – 'A Guide to HRT and the Menopause for Women in Lothian'. I am wondering why it is for just Lothian – is it different if you are a Glaswegian? I am distracted wondering how Weegies and Burgers would differ in their treatment so miss the next bit of the conversation – I reconnect just as she says having too high standards can sometimes be an issue for menopausal women. Clearly she hasn't seen the state of my home and doesn't know that I haven't ironed in 3 years and that I spent most of my working day yesterday on Facebook. But I nod and agree that it is a curse and I will try and lower my standards. This will mean no standards to be honest. But if that's what the Doctor orders! She recommends HRT patches and I agree. She runs through the risks but to be honest if I thought doing a deal with the local Junkies at the shopping mall would help the hell I am in then I'd do it. And I have done extensive research: I have watched famous menopausal women on telly and in OK magazine then checked if they took it. Well Davina McCall, Lorraine Kelly, Carol Vorderman & Andrea McLean all took it – and they all look fab and can string whole sentences together without forgetting what word comes next. (Yes I know this isn't proper scientific research but I feel it is an evidence based approach so good enough)

So Hot Flushes... Disturbed Sleep... Mood Swings... Chronic Tiredness... Joint Aches... BE GONE WITH YOU! Me and HRT will conquer.

As soon as I am brave enough to stick the first patch on...

CHAPTER 5

Holidaying with the menopausal girls

In this chapter, I bring to you – my meno-musings on holidays with other menopausal women.

Thirty years ago me and my pals had a fabulous holiday in Greece. So we've decided to do it all again!

And there are some changes! Twenty years ago our washbags bulged with cosmetics including the essential body shop face bronzer to contour those amazing cheekbones we all had but did not appreciate 'til the menopausal weight gain rendered them a distant memory! Now the essentials in our washbags are our tweezers! Not for our eyebrows as in a cruel twist of fate just as your chin gets hairier your eyebrows start to go bald!

Well, I say all of us. Mary Earhart hasn't got her tweezers as she was too tight to pay for her bag to go into the hold so they were confiscated as she took her carry-on bag through security. The security guard was rather shocked by her reaction. Clearly never having got between a menopausal woman and her tweezers before! I think Mary maybe over-reacted by screaming that if she was going to "blow the fucking plane up I would have brought a fucking grenade along not a pair of fucking tweezers"

But we managed to get her away before she could be arrested by a promise of gin and a lend of our tweezers when we got there! I had a quiet word with her about maybe restarting the HRT she gave up a couple of months ago.

We also have a shit load more medications. Thyroxine... statins... medication for high blood pressure all adorn the kitchen surfaces. And the HRT for some. Supplements for others. Personally, I can't see my symptoms being relieved by dabbing Aloe Vera on my temples but if it works for Shazza Austen then who am I to judge!

We have been splashing about in our bikinis in the pool. We worked out that between us we were about 14 stone heavier than last time but do you know how we managed to get bikini body ready? Yup... we just put a feckin bikini on... and 'ta dahhhh' that was it! Then we decided the seclusion of our villa meant an all over tan was a necessity. 'Suns oot taps aff' as they say in my home town! We are a little more battered than before with scars from ops and tumbles. And gravity has taken its toll. And we bear more emotional scars from the inevitable lows that join the highs of getting older... watching people we love get sick and die... divorces... heartbreaks... disappointments. So you'll excuse us for not giving a shit that the fashion journalists decree a one piece more flattering to the over 40 figure. We just follow the advice of this quote whose author remains anonymous – we 'look over each other's broken fences and admire the flowers in each other's gardens'

In the restaurants the waiters no longer ogle us... focussing instead on the young and the beautiful! But we wait patiently reflecting on our menopausal superpower of invisibility. We discount a bank heist but Fiona is with me on the shoplifting spree at John Lewis.

We wander off to our rooms and come back to ask what we went in for. We have conversations that are littered with "have I already said that?" And "am I repeating myself?" We are half way through our holiday books before we realise we think we have read them before.

It's definitely more SAGA than 18-30. Our reading glasses now adorn various surfaces and we take turns to lose them and help others find theirs.

We are gutted to realise we are so shit with technology we can't figure out how to get Strictly Come Dancing on the iPad. So we do our own version which owes more to enthusiasm than talent! But who cares coz we are not getting judged and no-one is watching ... we follow up with an X Factor competition with various cats that now live with us ever since the word got out that Shazza dropped a bit of chicken on the balcony last night yowling in accompaniment! But Simon can't hear us.

My friends Skype their kids – and I Skype Sweet Dog. We nap in the afternoon and go to bed at the same time we used to head out to the clubs at. And we don't care!

I am not sure if sunshine and being slightly pissed is helping our symptoms but they certainly help us give less of a toss about them!

CHAPTER 6

Returning home from holidays

In this chapter, I bring to you – my meno-musings on returning home from holidays.

In conclusion, holidaying on a Greek island suits the menopausal woman better than being at work. Indeed I feel there should be a 'Shirley Valentine' bill passed in parliament that all menopausal women should have 6 x 6 week holidays in the sun each year fully paid for.

The symptoms don't go when you are in the sun on holiday but they are so much easier to deal with. Menopausal exhaustion? Not a problem just have a kip on your sun lounger or head to the apartment for a wee siesta. Hot Flush? Jump into the pool to cool down. Become a Fat Bastard? No worries – Kaftans and flip-flops just don't care. And while being very slightly drunk all the time may not eliminate your symptoms it certainly makes you give less of a feck about them. But a week just isn't enough – it's just a tantalising glimpse of freedom before the chains of reality clip tightly round you again.

I remember loving the first day back at work after a holiday. Everyone admiring your tan and the lovely golden highlights in your hair. Showing off a couple of dreadlocks covered in bright string that you felt make you look cooler than cool and six or seven bright hippie friendship bracelets up one arm to complete the 'backfromholidays' look.

Not so much now. I went back last Wednesday. The pain started with getting up and tipping my half asleep body into the shower. Then I was drying my hair. And it was thick and claggy – and I am thinking what kind of fresh hell menopause symptom is this. Like thick butter was all through it. Then I had a thought... Did I rinse the conditioner off? Did I? OFFS – don't think so!! Menopausal Brain Fog! Back into the shower. Re-dry much happier hair though more orangey highlights than golden on account of old L'Oréal coloured locks not responding quite as well as natural young person hair. Sweet Dog annoyed as morning walk had to be cut short due to this disaster.

Then it is trying to put proper clothes on time. Clothes with waistbands... socks as well as proper shoes. I was lovely and smooth while away but now my legs and arms have a six o'clock shadow. They will have to stay that way as we are in October and as all women know – the razors go into hibernation 'til April – one benefit of Winter!

Clothes on – and carrying a few holiday pounds on top of the usual menopausal midriff makes me feel like I am in some kind of menopausal straitjacket.

And this isn't good when you are itching like feck! I think I was ranked number one in the 'tastiest human' section of the Greek MozzyTripAdvisor – I must have been as every Mozzy within a 500-mile radius came to dine on me. Feckin great – menopausal women are generally invisible but not to these annoying feckers who see me clearly as a feckin 'all you can eat' MozzyBuffet! So my 'not so golden tan' is peppered with angry red raised bumps.

However, I have a lovely emerald green long sleeved top that I think will show my slight tan off. I usually don't wear it as if I have a hot flush it shows sweat patches under my arms. But I got a great tip – incontinence pads are not just for protecting yourself from leaks when you sneeze – you can stick them under the arms of tops and they soak up the sweat! So I stick a couple under my arms and I am good to go.

Then into work – and amazingly I remember my password. I am ecstatic. Then my emails open and the agony replaces the ecstasy. It is said that around 200 billion emails are sent every day – and I feckin swear I am cc'd into every bloody one. I spend an hour hitting Delete... Delete... Delete...

Then menopausal rage hits as I see several with that highly offensive C word in it. It should not be allowed!

Yep – Christmas. Emails about Christmas leave/Christmas Nights Out/Christmas Secret Santa/fund for Christmas Decorations. It is October!!!! DELETE! DELETE! DELETE! I bang the keyboard with a fury only a menopausal woman can relate to. Jane tells me that she loves all the run up to Christmas and loves it starts so early. Well, I beg to feckin differ.

Then it is lunchtime. Baked potato with tuna in a large airless canteen just isn't the same as fresh seafood outside looking at the sea. And I am not sure how I going to get through the afternoon without at least half a carafe of white wine and a Rum Cocktail to wash it down.

Head to the loo and the mirror tells me that the beautician who promised me a hair free face for at least six weeks after charging me £90 for a full face threading was perhaps a little 'liar liar pants on feckin fire'. Desperate Dan looks sadly back at me – I get my trusty tweezers out to tackle the worst and wonder if I can budget in £90 a fortnight for the painful but effective threading. Nicola Sturgeon is putting sanitary protection in all schools and colleges and making it available for all low-income women to eradicate period poverty which is great. But I do think she may want to consider setting up places around Scotland to eradicate Menopausal Poverty. Hair removal, hair dye, incontinence pads, superduper tweezers, XL clothes; therapy; anger management classes; Botox; sunshine holidays – all free or at least at a massive discount. I'd vote in a politician that had something like this in their manifesto.

Back to the desk – my underarms feel funny. I check – one of the incontinence pads has gone! Oh no – I debate going to look for it. Then think feck it – no-one will know it is me. The stress gives me a hot flush and I now have a sweat patch under my right arm only. And my socks are really annoying me. Thankfully no meetings today as I think I am possibly incapable of speech.

I should probably do a bit of work... but maybe first I should just check out TravelZoo. Just to see what is there. Oh my goodness – what bargain end of season deals. I lift my phone to text my partner and suggest it. But then – what if they use factual evidence to dissuade me? Things like – we have no money left as we spent it all on rum cocktails/we said we would spend our next week off painting the spare room and looking for a second-hand wardrobe/ Christmas is coming up?

Probably best if I just book it and present it as a surprise. That will save a lot of debate and discussion. It is a complete bargain. And we will save money by not bothering with a wardrobe – guests can just use their suitcases as a wardrobe. And at Christmas, we will just watch that Kirstie Allsop thing and make our friends and family napkin holders out of discarded Sweet Dogs Chappie tins (or whatever she is doing this year). That will save another fair bit. I will need a few more clothes but the sales are on so will save a fortune there. Hair removal will cost a bit. But we can turn the heating off for the week which will pretty much save as much as we are spending give or take a few hundred quid. And maybe keep it off for a bit when we return – hot flushes keeping me cosy. Every cloud and all that.

CHAPTER 7

Do I look like I have slept well?

In this chapter, I bring to you – my meno-musings on menopausal insomnia.

3.16am. I am so sick of seeing those numbers on my clock. I used to see them often in my early 20s when I tumbled back from a nightclub and took a certain sense of pride at rocking home after 3am.

Now those numbers mock me – smugly telling me that once again I will have a sleepless night. And it is ironic that most of the day I suffer brain fog and forgetfulness. But for some reason between 3 and 4.30am, I can recall with total clarity every single mistake I have ever made in my life. And however tired I was when I went to bed – I will now be 100% wide awake.

Marlene Dietrich said it was the friends you can call at 4am that count. And this is potentially true. And I have a few that I probably could call at 4am. But only for emergencies – possibly of the kind involving something more critical than wanting to mull over the time that I took my trousers to the dry cleaners and when the man behind the counter shook them my pants with kitten print on them flew out of one of the legs and if maybe enough time has passed for me to go in again without being recognised. Or wanting to discuss the email I sent to the wrong person at work. Or any of the other mistakes I have made over the decades.

Without sleep, I transform from a grumpy ferocious fifty menopausal woman to a very tall 'terrible two' demonic toddler ready to let the world know I AM NOT HAPPY. And this is becoming an increasing problem lately due to changes at work. I can work from home a couple of days a week and so used to be able to fall back asleep at around 5 am and sleep 'til 8.50am then dash to my laptop and log on and join any conference calls from 9 am. This helped a lot – as opposed to the alternative of falling asleep at 5.30am then having to get up at half six to get ready for work and travel in.

I'd look a total mess but as only my Sweet Dog saw me (and she adores me and thinks I am the most beautiful person in the entire world even when I have fallen out of bed looking like a burst couch) it didn't really matter too much. I can sit with my hair matted and my old pyjamas and it is absolutely fine.

But then some feckin TechnoGeek at work discovered a way for us all to install cameras on our laptops and in the office – so we can 'see each other' when we are in different locations. And it was "virtually free so no real cost". The other TechnoGeeks were chuffed to bits about this and quickly set about installing the software. I, and other menopausal women along with other women that take more than 5 mins to be able to be seen without scaring small children were what you would call 'late adopters' of this technology. But then the three line whip came out – "you MUST have it installed – it is all lovely when we can all see each other"

Well, I beg to feckin differ! It is crap. In order to look presentable on the camera I must get up and look presentable in real life – from the waist up anyway. This takes at least 45 minutes – so forty-five minutes taken off my sleep is a LOT. It is also impossible when you are on camera to put the phone on speaker and mute and wander around putting washing on; dusting; doing a few sit-ups in an effort to be fit; flicking through a magazine; do your nails (and on one memorable day full of long conference calls repaint the entire hall) etc while you listen just enough to be able to make a sensible comment if your name is mentioned. AND you have to tidy up all the area around you as the camera captures that too and people judge... even if they say they don't... they DO! Jane thought it was funny to put a comment up on the screen about the chocolate wrappers on the dresser behind me but it so wasn't. Especially on four hours sleep. TBH nothing much was funny that day.

So at 3.30 am, I was stressing about whether or not I had switched the cooker off. You know what I mean? So I have to get up to check it – just in case. Then I got there and forget why I went downstairs. So I gave Sweet Dog a biscuit and head back upstairs only to remember the bloody cooker again. So back down again. Which means another biscuit for Sweet Dog and another chocolate biscuit for myself. Then I was wide awake.

Low testosterone is also a cause of poor sleep. I used to think testosterone was a man thing 'til I read a Health magazine that told me women actually produce more testosterone than oestrogen pre-menopause. And as levels decline when we hit the menopause, your sleep, your mood and your sex drive may also start to fall. Reduced levels of progesterone can also cause frequent waking and difficulty getting back to sleep. No shit Sherlock! The magazine did not give any feckin solutions to this state of affairs!!

And the days I can't work from home make the insomnia effects so much worse. Just as I am deep deep into the most wonderful sleep ever my alarm goes off (bloomin' same song that has woke me up for 6 years playing – was good for first few times but not I am sick of it and can't get it off my programmable alarm which cost a fortune so I just keep waiting 'til I can find someone to help me fix it and replace it with something a bit more current). Usually, I have a short internal debate and decide my hair isn't too bad – so decide to snooze for 20 mins as I've saved that time. Then it goes off again and I decide that I can just have a roll and sausage at work rather than make my porridge and fruit dish – so another 10 min snooze. Then I decide probably I can do my make up in the car at the traffic lights (not 100% sure if this is legal – Highway code says something about phones but makeup application they are less clear on) so another 10 mins.

I know it's bad when I got to work and Jane tells me about someone who has just been promoted because she 'slept her way to the top'. And I translated it into she was getting a good 8 hours sleep a night and was therefore shit hot at her job.

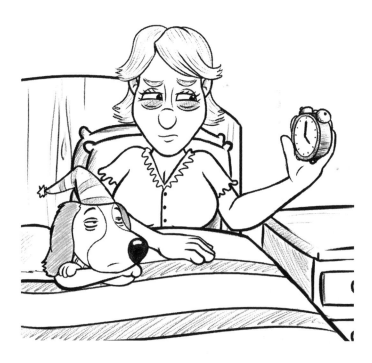

CHAPTER 8

A rant about women's magazines

In this chapter, I bring to you – a meno-rant on Women's magazines.

Imagine you were sitting on a sun lounger beside the pool and a woman came and sat beside you and started making comments to you about the people round the pool.

Comments like:

- Look at that fat girl over there – isn't she huge (about a woman who is at least 5 stone lighter than you!!)

- She has three kids by three fathers – it's terrible, isn't it!

- God would you look at her – so skinny you can see her ribs – it is gross, No wonder her husband left her

- OMG – did you see her dancing last night – total embarrassment

- See her – she is 60!! And I know for a fact she is shagging someone half her age

- Look at the cellulite on her arse!

- She really needs to get some work done on that face...

- We are all gonna gang up on that woman over there as she said something we don't like. She has apologised but we are gonna keep giving her a right kicking 'til we break her

- Look at her – she is SOOHHH not hot!

- That kid is right chubby – her mother is so skinny as well

- Can you believe someone with her belly is wearing a bikini!

- That woman over there was really fat – lost it all – and look at her now – put it all back on. Disgusting!

- Her over there – don't you think she is the worst dressed ever!

- Her over there – she tweeted that she and her husband fell asleep watching the telly – her marriage is clearly over!

- Her lip fillers haven't worked have they – or that boob job!

- See her – two weans and she is here on holiday without them. Left them with her husband – poor guy having to babysit.

She then snaps some pictures of the various women around the pool, taking and retaking 'til they are as unflattering as she can make them.

Finally, she offers you some vouchers for a slimming club, suggests you may want to change your hair as women over 40 should not have long hair and recommends you get botox and lip fillers. She departs with a few words on how you could look more youthful.

How would you feel? Uplifted? Good about yourself? Well, I would beg to feckin differ.

Because this is bullying/judging/mocking. It is not empowering in any way.

This happened to me on holiday. Except it wasn't a person – it was a pile of magazines left behind by a departing holidaymaker.

Who writes this shite? Sadly – it is women. Who edits it? Sadly – women again. And who buys it? Yep get that girl a prize – women again. Am I justified in this rant or am I just an old menopausal past it woman?

I mean have you ever seen FHM dedicate three pages to the size of Brad Pitts arse? Or Attitude show six pictures of Barack Obama and debate if he has gained a few pounds. Or Esquire line up some male pop artists and compare their thigh gaps? Nope – didn't think so.

Despite never having watched the Kardashians I could probably pick Kim's bare arse out of a line up before I'd recognise my own. And this pisses me off. As does the two-page article on the Strictly contestants – the write-ups on the males described their careers. The write-ups on the women described their clothes size/relationship status/shoe size and looks. I read about some celebrity apparently being cheap and desperate. You can argue that celebrities earn enough to put up with this and they can just pop to the cashpoint and press balance enquiry if they need cheering up. But it goes wider than that. What about all the young girls reading this. Reading this bullying/mocking/judging. These derogatory comments aimed at women just like them... tearing them apart and bashing them at every opportunity. Theresa May was described as a 'broken deckchair trying to unfold' – regardless of what you think of politics this is no way to describe any woman. What impact does this have on young woman's mental health?

With one in four now using self-harm as a coping mechanism – something has gone wrong.

These magazines do not speak for me and do not represent my views. I haven't bought them in years but as of now, I am boycotting their toxicity and their lazy journalism even if I see them on my regular trips to the Doctors Waiting room.

I think there is such a gap in the market for a new magazine. One that celebrates women's achievements – builds them up not breaks them down. Talks about things that matter to women everywhere. Good quality journalism. I even have a name – Avid. The reverse of 'Diva'.

And never ever mention diets and bikini bodies.

CHAPTER 9

Visiting the Menopause Café

In this chapter, I bring to you – my meno-musings on visiting Menopause Cafés.

One Saturday a few months ago, I went to a Menopause Café (also known as a Rest and Rant – Restaurant… geddit?). They are currently running throughout the UK with the objective of 'increasing awareness of the menopause Café on those experiencing it, their friends, colleagues and family'.

I was a little apprehensive. My Aunt Gill has been pushing for me to go to a Menopause Commune where women rub oil into each other's feet and exchange stories on their menopause journey. They then recite poetry and sing supportive songs while standing in a healing circle. They all bring presents for each other apparently that demonstrate their journey. She even offered to make me a fabric heart with a little tear that had been sewn back up to represent my vulnerability to take along as my gift (she thought it might be the lack of a present that made me so reluctant!!! I had to beg to feckin differ and explain I would rather experience a 10 hour hot flush with urinary incontinence and heart palpitations than go to that kind of event).

My friend Tina the Turner (her name is actually Tina Ciccone but her moniker has come about due to her remarkable ability to convert straight women to lesbianism) said she wanted to come to. I was surprised tbh – didn't really think it was her thing – but she explained that she was single again and thought it would be a good opportunity to 'meet some lovely new women'.

I am not sure if the organiser would appreciate their event being used as a kind of face to face Menopausal Tinder – but who are we to judge?

She is also looking at potential venues for her 50th and as the Menopause Café was being held at Dumfries House in Ayrshire which is on her list of options she had two good reasons to go. Me – well they had me at 'free biscuits and cake'.

We did discuss the possibility of it being utterly depressing with a few sad women eating those cakes that made of beetroot and avocado and so are not really cakes. We worried we would have nothing in common with them apart from more than a passing interest in incontinence pad adverts. I also Googled the background of the Café – and found out that they are based on Death Café's where people get together to talk about dying which didn't really increase our enthusiasm. So we arranged a 'get out' plan of having to leave after an hour 'to pick the kids up'. Then if it was crap we could disappear but if it was good we would pretend that a neighbour had offered to take them.

We needn't have worried – it was brilliant. Not just the cakes (though they were good!!) but very well organised with a fabulous facilitator. She was unflappable even when the lift jammed and a ladder had to be dropped down and hot grumpy menopausal women had to be hauled out one at a time by a team of strong willing volunteers (not me obvs – one benefit of being a menopausal fatty is that no-one asks you to help with physical activities – Result!).

Tina was a bit raging as she saw a few gorgeous women and she hadn't worn her hair extensions or makeup or false nails as she felt she wouldn't fit in if she was too glamorous. We all had a good laugh though – discussing symptoms with the group – and what worked/didn't work for us. We also found out that there is a 6-week course being run at the Centre. Tina became very inter-ested when she heard Camilla Parker Bowles gynae comes up to do consultations during the 6 weeks. Camilla is her ultimate girl crush. We are not sure if this is just a rumour but the Centre was set up by Prince Charles – so who knows? In any case, I doubt Camilla would be accompanying him – but I am not into bursting bubbles so didn't say anything.

We were having such fun that we totally forgot about our 'kids excuse' so we looked a bit blank when the facilitator brought it up. On reflection, it was a silly excuse as we don't have kids and both suffer from menopausal brain fog. There were a few social workers there that looked a bit disapproving but I think we got away with it.

I would definitely recommend it – I got a lot from it and left feeling happy and uplifted. The cakes are really good too. And Tina is taking one of the ladies we met out for lunch on Tuesday so it seems to have panned out alright for her too.

I went back again a few weeks later alone as Tina was all loved up and none of my other friends admit to being menopausal. I would definitely recommend and not just for the free cake (though there is a very varied selection and they don't mind how many slices you eat) and the goody bag (lots of nice things in there including chocolate and a little packet of love hearts in the last one).

Bit of advice though – put your glasses on and look carefully at the packaging of the treats in these goody bags – I spent 20 mins with my face covered in lube as the pack closely resembled a free face pack sample. I did notice the YES VM in big font but didn't read the small print and thought VM was maybe Visage Mask or something – turns out it was Vaginal Moisturiser!!

To be fair it actually did quite a good job – my skin looked really good and glowing. And I suppose if it is sensitive enough to be used down there then it will be fine on your face. But don't think I will be making a habit of it.

The conversation at my Menopause Café table turned to a heated debate over what was the worst menopausal symptom. I cannot recall what we decided the worst one was but let's face it – there are quite a few to choose from. The Menopausal Fairy really is a gift that just keeps giving.

I was making use of the bright sunlight this morning by positioning the mirror in the sunniest window and plucking out the hairs from my chin and for the first time also my neck which was an odd experience and trying to remember what we agreed the worst symptom was. There were a couple that complained about the excess hair that comes from the fluctuating hormones but that isn't the worst for me. I mean – if it wasn't for my supply of tweezers and focussed attention I would resemble that bearded lady in The Greatest Showman (apart from the singing bit because I can't hold a note) but it just takes a bit of work and it is generally fine. I was going to tell these women that as they were visibly hirsute but I managed to restrain myself which is unusual – as many women will testify the filter between brain and mouth often goes missing during the menopausal years

The hot flushes were keenly debated – if you haven't had one you just can't imagine it – after my first few I was Googling 'spontaneous human combustion' as I seriously thought I might be a candidate for it – because I just could not believe that that level of heat in your body was natural and normal under any circumstances. But I am pretty sure that came second in the list of crap symptoms.

The menopausal midriff is a bit crap too but that is what smocks, loose tops and pregnancy jeans are for.

The anxiety – the continual worry! My boss asked me to check the temperature of Tenerife while we were going to be away on a work jolly otherwise known as a Strategy Weekend. I pointed out that that it was 24 degrees when we go there then strangely went up by one degree each day we were there. Jane kindly pointed out I was looking at the dates rather than the temperatures. I have regular 3am mortification episodes over that one.

That bone-crushing exhaustion that hits you like a ten-ton truck when you least want it to. That exhaustion that pulls down on every bone and every fibre of your being when you just have to lie down before you fall down. When you truly can't believe you can keep going for another minute.

Its seems like there are ten million celebrities currently banging on about their 'terrible menopause' and how they solved it my spending ten million quid at a Harley Street Doctor and taking 2 years off work and just resting, going on retreats, having a personal chef whip them up lovely plant-based meals and a personal trainer to keep them in shape – and recommending we all do the same – kind of gets on my tits a bit. And certain celebrities kindly organising a big conference that we can go to for just £95 or £150 if we want the VIP package – I mean did they forget a feckin pension plan or something so decided to make a few quid by re-inventing themselves to Menopause Advocate (I mean who would advocate the feckin menopause ffs)... I know that's not really a symptom but it pisses me off so I am going to include it. Feck off with your glossy hair and your slim bodies and perfect skin – feck off, feck off, feck off – stop telling us all how we can be just like you. We can't – we don't have millions of quid and if we don't show up at work for two years we'll end up on the streets selling the Big Issue – which to be fair would stop us worrying about the menopause I suppose?

Anyway, I digress – and I have just remembered. The worst symptom – forgetfulness!! Or at least that is the worst for me. Everyone is different but this is certainly the one that has the biggest impact on my life. I could write for hours on the various episodes that have blighted me since the Menopausal Fairy decided to raid my memory but here are a few highlights:

- One morning I was walking back from the Supermarket convinced I had forgotten something. I had made a list but I had forgotten it – so had to rely on memory. I ran through the things in my head – bread, bananas, eggs, bacon (not doing the vegan thing anymore), and washing powder. Racked my brains. Got home, made a cup of tea and a bacon sandwich. Then I realised there was no slavering dog trying to get a bit – the dog!!! OMG I had forgotten Sweet Dog. Sweet Dog was still tied up outside Tesco waiting for her rubbish useless owner. Oh dear... that dog already has abandonment issues (she is a rescue) what have I done I had to leap in the car and tear down to find her like Naebodys Wean – patiently waiting but with a sadness in her eyes that made me cry my eyes out all the way home. It made me think of Greyfriars Bobby and that made me cry even more. Forgetting is awful but then remembering you forgot is even worse.

- The other night I stood clicking my car key at the door getting increasingly frustrated it wasn't opening. Then realised I was trying to open my front door. Thank goodness none of my neighbours witnessed that debacle.

- Last week at work I could not remember where I had parked the car. Our car park is HUGE and goes on literally for miles and I could not remember the section I had left it in. I wandered round pressing the key button hopefully looking out for the flashing lights. Nothing. Finally, in frustration, I decided to get the bus back home then return late at night when it would be the only feckin car left and easy to spot. So I waited at the bus stop... Then remembered – I'd got the feckin bus in that morning as I was going out for a drink with a friend. Which I had also forgotten but at least remembered in time to still make the by then much-needed bottle of Sauvignon Blanc.

- Another day I went to someone's desk at work to ask something and when I got there I hadn't a clue what I went to ask. And just stood looking at them like some weird stalker. I have lost track of the number of times I have stared blankly at my screen trying to remember what the feck the password is... that blinking cursor mocking me as I try to remember if I made a note of it anywhere and if so what it was.

- Panicking that I had lost my mobile and hunting through my bag for it – then telling my mum I would have to go to look for it. And she kindly pointed out I was actually talking on her on it, therefore, it must be in my hand.

Yet oddly I can remember all the lyrics to almost every 80s Top Ten hit! And many of the dance steps which I have taught Sweet Dog so we can partner each other dancing round the kitchen.

CHAPTER 10

A brief history of the menopause

In this chapter, I bring to you – my meno-musings on the history of the Menopause.

It's not really been that long since we didn't ever have to think of the menopause as most of us would have kicked the bucket before it happened. I was thinking what it might be like for previous generations who didn't have the access to the (still limited) information we have. So I am trying to think of some positives of us over our mothers and grandmothers. I've thought and thought and thought 'til my head hurts.

I thought about it when I was in a traffic jam this morning. But then noticed some black hairs on my chin and I had to get going with my tweezers. (I have tweezers in my car, in my handbags, in my make-up bags – and next to every mirror in the house. I will not leave home without them. I will not be like Mrs Christie at school who we all laughed at with her whiskers and wiry beard) Fluctuating hormones brought these lovely wee additions to my face about 9 months ago (said no-one ever!!). In bright light, you will see them in menopausal women's faces – springing out of nowhere. But don't under any circumstances point it out to them – trust me on that one! I mean, I'd rather know, but turns out my friend would rather have stayed ignorant when I mentioned her hairy whiskers in a genuine effort to be helpful. I would recommend simply buying a magnifying mirror for birthdays/Christmases as an alternative to the direct approach. You never want to piss a menopausal woman off. Like ever!

So I do some research and we are lucky – honestly. We are so much luckier than our great great great grannies. In those days the menopause was known as the 'gateway to death'. Not any more – we can often have a third, maybe even half our lives left when it is over. To be fair we will spend it fat, knackered, a bit bald, hairy-faced and highly irritable. But it's still better than the alternative.

It was Aristotle who first mentioned the menopause. And this was about 300BC. Maybe he should have spent as much time looking at this than he did teaching Alexander the Great and we may have been so much further forward in terms of treatment. But he couldn't really be arsed so limited his work on the menopause to declaring it a time when women got 'colder and drier'. Hmmm – Aristotle had clearly never lay in bed with a woman having a hot flush otherwise he would have been more likely to have declared something along the lines of 'for Christ's sake – you are literally melting my feckin skin' which is a regular declaration from my bed partner while rolling to the furthest end of the bed and dramatically fanning the covers for air. Sometimes I really do prefer Sweet dog who doesn't mind at all and clambers merrily onto my tummy when it happens – think she sees it as a massive hot water bed to have fun on.

But after Aristotle, no-one really bothered about the menopause much 'til the mid-1800s. Possibly because not many women lived much past 40 for much of the intervening years. So if you did – it was probably like winning the lottery.

It was 1823 when a French physician coined the phrase 'menopause' meaning ceasing of the month. The first medications were not quite the plethora we have on offer now. In the 1800s cannabis was prescribed. This would have been a preferred option given some of the alternatives – douche of lead, morphine and chloroform anyone? What about testicular juice? Or the filtered juice of a guinea pigs ovaries. I may send these examples in to Ant and Dec for the food challenges in the next I'm a Celeb! Or what about a clitoridectomy (yes that is what you think it is) as recommended by influential surgeon Baker Brown. Or bloodletting (some doctors felt it was because women no longer passing blood that triggered the symptoms – so if they took blood out regularly it would 'fix' them) Leeches were attached often to genitalia to assist with such treatment (in those days Doctors were nearly all men – I'll say no more...)

In 1855 Lawson Tait, who was an influential physician, considered menopausal women to be in grave danger of mental derangement and incurable dementia. I can't blame him – I thought the same when the symptoms started, and so did many people who know me. But his treatment which was simply to lock them up in asylums seems a little extreme. The guy also believed Jack the Ripper was a woman... so perhaps his theories should have been discounted then...

The Purity Movement Writers declared a bad experience of the menopause to be a sign of sin – and said that it showed the woman had been badly behaved when young. Yes – maybe – but I have some great memories to look back on during my sleepless nights – none of them involving working out at the gym with some tofu and sparkling water for dinner!

Moving on through the years it didn't get much better. Menopause is now a popular topic particularly on Women's Hour (my fave radio programme). However, when first mentioned on radio in 1948, there was a massive outcry – 'lowering of broadcasting standards' and 'acutely embarrassing' were two of the many complaints.

In 1966, Dr Robert Wilson declared us all 'galloping catastrophes'. The phrase I reclaimed for this book and for myself. I love the thought of being a 'galloping catastrophe' Better than being a galloping apostrophe which is what I thought it said when I first read it (after a couple of glasses of wine). 'Move out of the way please, galloping catastrophe coming through'. Love it!!

The topic is no longer taboo – and we have much more information, support and choice of treatment than so many of our female ancestors. I think laughing at yourself and with others on some of the more ridiculous symptoms with a bottle or three of wine is something our grannies and probably our mothers would never have done. And were probably the worse for it.

So from one Galloping Catastrophe to another. Let's celebrate the fact we have come a long long way and make our third act count!

CHAPTER 11

Speccy four-eyes

In this chapter, I bring to you – my meno-musings on discovering that as well as being menopausal and all the associated crap symptoms – I am also half blind.

The joys of getting older just keep coming! Dodgy Knee, Arthritic Finger, Sore Lower Back and Short Term Memory Loss all come out in force to welcome Dodgy Eyesight.

The optician's diagnosis was not a complete surprise. For a few months I have had to inch the menu in restaurants further and further from my face. I have to finally concede that my arms are not long enough to keep going with this strategy. I'd also dialled in to the wrong conference calls at work, having not been able to read the number properly.

I did find out some great gossip though as it took about 15 mins before the conference call organiser realised they had a cuckoo in the nest (clearly I was not going to drop off as soon as I realised... this is the closest I have come to being a fly on the proverbial and it was intoxicating). (PA – soz team but Vanessa was right – the ten zillionth restructure of the year is on its way).

But of course, it could not be as simple as just a pair of reading glasses. Turns out I am long and short-sighted so need two bloody pairs. I didn't even know that was possible!! And twice the bloody expense. I had kind of guessed though – driving was becoming an issue especially at night, with the cars all merging into soft amber lights ahead and behind.

The deciding factor was running as fast as I could to platform 6 for my train and leaping on it, only to hear the announcer declare it was going in completely the opposite direction. WTF – I leapt off quickly and berated the Railway guard about wrong platform information. He kindly pointed out that my train was on Platform 8 – then more smugly than kindly pointed out I had just missed it!! Had to wait another hour which meant breaking my attempt at being sugar free again (I really do want to give up sugar but for just a pound I can get almost ten minutes of sheer happiness with a Family Sized Galaxy... if anyone can tell me what brings more happiness for a pound then I am all ears (so far Deafness hasn't joined my 'getting old party' but give it time).

So £800 quid later (coz no other speccy four-eyes fecker told me just to get the prescription and go on the internet for much cheaper glasses until after I had coughed out to a rather surprised but happy optician – of course since doing that every bloody specky four-eyes has told me. Horse. Stable Door. Bolted. Anyone?), I left with two pairs of glasses and an urge to spend more cash. Having spent £800, another £80 on a handbag seemed a snip. And I did need a bigger one now that I have two pairs of glasses to keep in them. I remember the days of youth where I would head out with one small bag with cash and a Body Shop strawberry lip gloss. With each passing decade, my bag gets bigger. As well as glasses, I now have tweezers, small magnifying mirror to use when using the tweezers (just as an aside – either those bloody hormonal chin bristles have doubled overnight or my glasses plus magnifying mirror are a reflection of the bearded lady everyone else has been seeing when they have looked at me); water bottle (which is always heavy as I keep forgetting to drink the recommended 2 litres); diary (coz I forget everything and can't figure out the calendar thing on my phone); a notepad (to write things that I need to remember – coz if not written down now – it ain't happening); tissues (to mop up the sweats); nuts and seeds so I don't binge on chocolate; chocolate wrappers coz I don't really like nuts and seeds very much; tampons all the time coz the days of being regular as clockwork are well gone. So with all of this and the glasses – a much larger bag is a necessity rather than a luxury. And it can almost be described as a medical purchase as it assisted with the depression as yet another part of my body gives up.

So I rock up at work with my fab new bag (after driving halfway with this bloody annoying beeping in the car and not knowing what it was – then finally working out the stupid car thought my bag was a person and wanted me to put its seatbelt on). It's not that heavy ffs. So I had to push it onto the floor to stop it – and of course, all my crap fell out all over the footwell). I fish out my specs and am feeling happy coz I am now seeing them as a fashion statement.

One of my colleagues Alan looks at me, head tilted to the side. 'They are OK' he says 'but you do look better when you don't wear them'.

'You look better when I don't wear them too!' I responded, internally giving myself a high five for such a witty reply – with brain fog these are few and far between. My satisfaction with this is short lived as he turns back to his spreadsheet. I resolve to use this line again in the future though but not with people who look at spreadsheets all day.

'They are cute' laughs Jane, looking up from her spreadsheet. 'You look a bit like a Harry Potter'

I don't laugh, partly because a 12-year-old boy wizard was not the image I was aiming for when I paid £500 for these particular designer glasses – and also because she didn't laugh at my earlier witty comment.

So after three days of being a glasses wearer, I have to conclude it may take some time to acclimatise to them. I used to like lying on my side in bed reading – try doing that with specs! They dig right into your head and ear. So have to sit up with a shawl now looking like my old Granny. I can't drink hot tea when I am reading as they steam up.

And they are never bloody clean. I wipe them constantly but always there is a mark. Yesterday I was ready to go to the Doctors convinced I had glaucoma but it was just a fingerprint on the (twice cleaned) lens.

I don't need them all the time – so when I am not reading at work I stick them on top of my head in what I consider a rather intellectually fetching way, but then I forget and lean forward and they fall off which spoils the effect.

And what is with people wanting to 'try them on' then making comments about how blind I must be. I am sure this is against one of our disability policies. I mean, you couldn't ask someone to borrow their wheelchair and talk about how crap their legs must be without HR sending you on a four-day Diversity course. And then Big Fat Freda McCall borrowed them and gave them back with the arms all stretched. I am a fatso too but so far my head has not increased in size so I had to mould them back into my face shape. She has tiny feet though – I am tempted to ask to try her shoes on and stretch them all to buggery. See how she likes it. But she does have a bit of an odour problem there so I probably won't. Don't want to add smelly feet and verruca's to my problems. Actually – my feet are really good with no problems at all now that I think of it. Probably due to giving up on heels and living in sensible sketchers for the last 3 years helping there.

But you gotta laugh. Coz where would you be without a sense of humour?

Working opposite me on spreadsheets probably!

CHAPTER 12

Menopause at work policy

In this chapter, I bring to you – my meno-musings on menopause at work policies.

My pal Tina sent me her company's recently developed 'Menopause Policy'. 'How enlightened!' I thought. Until I read it. Six pages of twaddle with only one meaningful tangible item of support. Well, when I say meaningful – I mean 'menopausal women can be offered a fan as long as it is environmentally friendly'. That was it!! Clearly, they had not actually consulted with any menopausal women otherwise I feel the policy may have looked very different!

So as a free gift to all the HR and High Heid Yins out there – I have developed meaningful Menopause guidance that you are welcome to copy and paste into your existing HR policy documentation – saving you time and money that you can spend on providing free wine to Menopausal Women at the end of each shift.

Here we go...

Menopausal Women at Work: A guide for Managers

Introduction

The menopause can affect how a woman performs her work and her relationships with colleagues. For example she just may not want to be arsed working sometimes particularly if she has been up all night with hot flushes. She may also often refer to her colleagues using such terms as 'Dicktard', 'Fuckwit' and even the C word. It is imperative therefore that 'reasonable adjustments' are made to accommodate her needs at this time.

Guidance

All managers must adhere to the following guidance:

Cases of minor misconduct or unsatisfactory performance is best ignored. If, using the case above as an example, the menopausal woman does refer to a colleague in a derogatory tone then pause to consider if she is perhaps justified and that colleague is indeed a twat. Indeed you may want to use this opportunity to remove all fucktards from your team as hormones can mean that the menopausal women can be prone to actions that may see her end up in prison and this is to be avoided at all costs. Honesty is one of the benefits you can reap from a menopausal woman. If you want honest 360-degree feedback then rather than refer to the made up crap your subordinates write just in case you can track it back to them – simply ask the menopausal woman. It is imperative that you foster a safe environment for the woman to say exactly what they think.

If, after careful consideration, you do decide that action must be taken against the menopausal woman in these cases we would suggest a paid day off or bottle of wine as potential acceptable responses. Such kindness will be appreciated but possibly responded to with tears of gratitude so ensure you have tissues ready just in case.

More serious cases such as posting 'XYZ company is full of twats and arseholes' on social media or punching a colleague in the face are probably due to mitigating circumstances such as hormonal fluctuations and perhaps self-medicating with wine and gin. Therefore the usual social media rules will be relaxed for the menopausal woman. Indeed the firewalls will be removed from their logons to enable them to talk on Support Forums when they feel the need and to order expensive shoes if they feel that is necessary as both can be a great support at this time of change.

Central to this policy is the ownership of temperature control – it should be handed entirely over to the menopausal woman. If others in the office complain that it is too cold then they should be asked to wear a jumper. It is imperative that the menopausal woman is able to regulate the temperature around her as there is fuck all she can do about the raging inferno inside her. If budget permits then for a fee, Sam Heughan and/or Helen Mirren can be employed to waft large palm leaves as and when required.

Headphones and access to carefully selected Spotify playlists will be provided with tissues in case they cause a hormonal woman to become emotional when they realise every line means something – nothing by Adele as it might make them sob uncontrollably and nothing by Eminem as it might make them angry. A focus group will be created to come up with acceptable songs for inclusion This Girl is on Fire and Hot Stuff are two examples of tunes that may be suitable.

If the menopausal woman is expected to wear a uniform then it must be able to be adapted. If she would prefer to wear a loose smock with Birkenstocks rather than pour herself into a tight skirt and blazer then this should be accommodated. Indeed, she may choose to simply come to work in her pyjamas and this should not be discouraged as it is entirely appropriate at this time of life. A bra is unlikely to be worn – not in a sexy Kardashian way but more in a 'tits swinging round the waist' kind of way – and this should be considered totally appropriate.

Exceptional circumstances should be considered and responded to appropriately. For example, a menopausal woman may find it beneficial to just piss off from everyone and everything and sit on a beach in Greece either to write bad poetry by herself or to shag the waiter like in Shirley Valentine. Every menopausal woman is different so there is no structured guidelines around this but we would suggest a 3-month menopausal career break on full pay as a minimum standard to aim for. This leave may not be shared with a partner even if they beg – it isn't about them. They can sort their own manopause out (if you haven't heard of it it's a bit like man flu but with motorbikes)

Fully flexible working will be encouraged as it is very likely that the menopausal woman will only find a cure for her insomnia three seconds before the alarm goes off. So it is best if she can simply hit the off button and return to sleep 'til she feels able to come in. Or just work at home watching Loose Women if she feels that would be a more supportive environment.

Sweet Dogs will be given as 'therapy dogs' to any woman who feels she needs them.

Organisations would be well advised to review their benefits and perks policy. It is a cruel truth that as the menopausal woman's eyesight starts to deteriorate their facial hair will start to increase. Laser eye surgery should, therefore, be offered as a tax-free benefit as well as high-quality tweezers. Incontinence pads should join the sanitary protection in the toilets and vodka should join the chocolate in the vending machines. Note – JOIN – not replace.

Mandatory training will be given to managers to help them implement this policy (unless the manager is a menopausal woman in which case she can have the day off to lie beside the river and read magazines and drink those wee cans of Pimms you get in Tesco. There will be pre-course work – which is likely to involve being kept awake all night by an incessant chatter in your ear about every little thing you ever did wrong or messed up in your life. You will need to dress in your warmest vest and coat then twice in the night your electric blanket will be turned to full and you can make a decision whether to just lie in it or get up and change fully before experiencing the same thing two hours later. The next day you will attend a full day's immersion session to enable you to fully empathise with the menopausal woman. Such sessions are not restricted to, but will likely include: standing in front of an industrial oven on full blast for 15 mins 4 times during the day to develop empathy for the hot flush – followed by being put in a sealed room with lots of midgies to feel that unbearable itching. A temporary full frontal lobotomy will be given at the end of the course and not reinstated for 24 hours so the manager can experience brain fog and forgetfulness at first hand. Additional places will be made available for husbands and partners where required. It is recognised that additional training in conflict resolution may be required and this will be an optional module that we believe most managers will choose to take up.

We believe these measures set the tone for a positive working environment for the menopausal woman. To ensure the long term success of this policy any transgressions will be dealt with by a forum of menopausal woman headed by Big Mags who is permanently hangry due to trying to get rid of the menopausal midriff but this keeps her focussed on the importance of dealing with any infringements of due process.

Menopausal ambassadors will be around to help where required, with stocks of hankies; numbers for therapists (six sessions provided free of charge); vouchers for plus size stores; wine; chocolate and access to the menopause room which is equipped with cool comfortable beds that rock you gently to sleep when you need it most.

The End

Managers and Companies Everywhere – you are WELCOME! No charge – simply make a donation of a bottle of wine or gin or large box of chocolates to the next menopausal woman you meet.

CHAPTER 13

My Magnetic Growler

In this chapter, I bring to you my menopausal musings on my Fanny Magnet. This was something I bought when I decided I would not take anything internally for the menopause. It is essentially two magnets that you put on your knickers and apparently it 'may' help with hot flushes, bloating, mood swings and fatigue. The packaging also says it 'may' help with improved skin tone, sleep and libido. The words 'may' appear a lot.

I bought mine when on the way to meet my 'good time pal' Rosie Alcott – better known as 'Five Pint Rosie' (on account of the fact everyone counts the beers she drinks when out and makes an excuse to leave when she hits pint number five as she then transforms from a lovely kind person to a mental case who wants to fight anyone within a 100 yard radius). My work bestie Jane swears by it. It was £35 quid in Boots and the sales assistant who located it for me advised me that I should do HRT as she used it and it gave her back her sex drive which I did think was maybe too much information to divulge when we had barely met. But I got 140 boots advantage points and I am not convinced I want to take drugs yet so am giving it a go.

I opened it up in the loo in the pub and carefully put it on the front of my knickers as instructed. It is a lovely purpley glittery colour. Then I went to meet Rosie for lunch in the same pub feeling most grown up. I am taking control of my symptoms. She finally arrived and leant forward to give me a hug. As she did so – her lovely long metal pendant swung forward and attached itself to my groin!! She yanked it off 'what the fuck' she said. I explained my magnet and we got out the instructions. It is a 'powerful static magnetic device'. She had some nail scissors in her bag – we tried attaching them and a spoon. The spoon didn't hold but the nail scissors did!

She asked how much it was as she might get one for her kids Christmas. I told her and she said 'what the fuck?' again and told me she had a ton of crap fridge magnets the kids had collected over the years and she would have gladly given me them for free. She texted her husband to tell him, a bit pissed off coz I would not let her photograph it to put on Instagram. He replied saying he was changing my name in his phone to 'Magneto Growler'. My pal thought this hysterical. I, to be honest, was less amused. After a few glasses of wine, I started finding it funnier. And we found all manner of metal objects to attach to my groin – each one funnier than the last. I finally headed for home a little worse for wear.

I felt worse than I thought I would the morning after. I normally go for lunchtime drinking where possible as the hangover then takes place when you are asleep thus leaving you refreshed for the next day. But I felt like I had been hit by a bus. I read a bit more of the instructions of the magnet. Apparently, the only side effect is 'slight flu-like symptoms' in the first couple of days. Well as today has gone on I have felt worse and worse. Could be co-incidence as everyone and his dog has a bug of some sort just now. But am not feeling good with swollen glands, sore throat, runny nose and thick head. Also – you are supposed to wear it 24/7 – I don't really like wearing knickers at night. But it won't stay on otherwise. Who knows – this might be all I need.

I consider this the next day as I queue for my morning coffee. But then I realised I had a pair of tweezers attached to my crotch. FFS. I had dropped them in the car when I saw a police car (the mobile phone legislation is pretty clear but the use of tweezers while in control of a car is less so and I wasn't taking any risks). And my bloomin' fanny magnet which attracts anything metal within 100 feet had decided to take them hostage. Then at lunchtime my groin is pulled towards the metal of the conveyer belt and I thrust forward like a blooming female Harvey Weinstein!

CHAPTER 14

Another visit to the doctor

In this chapter, I bring to you – my meno-musings on going to the Doctors when you are menopausal and poorly

So I WAS poorly. Very poorly. I am getting most reluctant to visit the Doctor because of my previous ailments I had self-diagnosed – all of which I was tested for and found negative for. All my ailments ended up being symptoms of the menopause and so at that point I had determined only to visit the Doctor if it was really serious so that I would not get a reputation for being a hypochondriac and potentially cause them to miss something in a sort of 'girl who cried wolf' kind of way.

But I can barely move. I am existing on a diet of Lemsips and phish food ice cream (medicinal as it is the only thing that will ease my throat). My head hurts, my chest is congested, my eyes have disgusting excretions coming from then. My ear is on fire. My body is on fire and I am sweating (though that could be the flushes – it is kind of hard to tell).

So I call the receptionist. I tell her I am not sure whether or not to come in – I might be wasting the Doctors time. She listens to my fragile voice describing my awful symptoms and I hear her tapping away at her computer. I am hoping she is looking at my file and not ordering something off Amazon as she is very quiet.

'I think you should come in' she says 'I can get you an emergency appointment at 2pm'.

I take it. Then I start to panic. It must be serious if they have fitted me in on the same day. Menopausal anxiety, sickness and Google are a troublesome combination. A few clicks and I realise I have symptoms of pleurisy. Or maybe pneumonia. I wonder if I should pack a small bag in case they send me straight to hospital. A few more clicks and I suspect I may have a lung abscess. Maybe chronic bronchitis. Or even chronic obstructive pulmonary disease!!

I am really panicking now and start to work out how long I can live for if I have to give up work to recover. I am kicking myself for not taking out income protection cover. That starts me worrying about whether I have mortgage protection cover – will they let me remortgage or do interest only payments? I logon to see the pitiful amount of savings I have and deduce I could last about 5 weeks and 2 days before I would be out on the street. Sweet Dog may have to downgrade to a supermarket own brand dogmeat!

Then it's time to go. In my younger days, in the very rare event I went to a Doctor, I only ever went if I wanted a sick note so I could skive off work (I have realised though that as I get closer to 50 then Doctors/Medical Practitioners take you much more seriously than when I was 22 and the bloody Doctors would shush me away with no sick note and some advice to 'cheer up'). I worry and worry on the way there – Receptionists are trained to pick out malingerers so she must have realised I am very much at risk

I go in and answer the usual questions – smug as always with the no smoking... less smug with the units of alcohol per week. No sign of scales, thank God, as that would have wiped the smugness completely off my face.

I panic as I realise I have no bra on – feck – what if she wants to listen to my chest. As she checks temperature, oxygen flow, etc., I get more and more anxious – what will she think if I have to remove my top and my boobs are thrust into her face? She might put something in my notes that I am a total loony (if it isn't there already?)

She listens to my back with her stethoscope thing. She gets me to cough and I do a delicate little cough. She asks again – then tells me to do a full on deep cough. God, she is a Doctor of a certain age – I am a menopausal women – does she not get why I am coughing so lightly? But I obey and hope for the best – fortunately it is only a little bit of wee that comes out and I think I get away with it. I cough again and again for her – it starts to get quite traumatic – my bladder is really full from all the Lemsips. She stops there – doesn't do my chest – maybe coz she can see from that there is no bra and doesn't want to risk it.

'Just a cold', she says.

'I beg to feckin differ', I say.

'Yes', she says, 'lots of it about'.

Does she not realise just how sick I am? I panic and worry again that maybe she was too embarrassed to listen to my braless chest and maybe that would have been the decider in sending me to the hospital for immediate treatment. Maybe she has seen all of the appointments for last year and a 'hypochondriac' note on my file.

'Antibiotics?' I croak. 'Oh no', she says. 'Two paracetamol every four hours, fluids and rest – you'll be fine'. Well again, I beg to feckin differ – it will serve her right if I have to be blue lighted into A&E at 3am with one of the many illnesses I clearly have.

So I return home to bed, picking up some more phish food ice cream with paracetamol on the way back. I try to buy three packs but am told that I can only buy 2 – apparently if you buy more than that you are probably planning to kill yourself and the supermarket refuses to potentially be a guilty party in such an arrangement. I resist the urge to say 'FFS – if I really wanted to top myself do you think I wouldn't just choose another method or just simply pop to another shop' but it is hard as I am due a rant. No need though – as she tells me she'll just put it through on another transaction and that will solve it.

Next day I suspect I might be getting slightly better. I truly think you can judge how sick you are by how interesting you find daytime telly. Yesterday Sweet Dog and I were desperate to find out if that lovely man on Jeremy Kyle was indeed that poor girl's father and was hooked for the DNA results. Today I am couldn't care less if the man the lady wants to marry may be her cousin. I mean I record it – coz I want to find out. But I don't watch it.

I may actually be getting better! But I am now obsessed with the various 'diagnose your own illness' websites there are – and I may need to make another visit to the Doctors soon.

I may change surgery first though...

CHAPTER 15

Summertime and the menopause ain't easy

In this chapter I bring to you – my musings on being a menopausal woman in the summertime.

We had our Scottish Summer on Saturday morning. Summer as a menopausal woman is, shall we say, a little more challenging than summer as a non-menopausal woman.

It started well – I did wake early which is unusual. I am a little ragey as my partner is away so I cannot blame his snoring for waking me up.

Early waking is a problem for the menopausal woman... sleep is oh so precious at this 'time of change'. But Bastarding birds do not respect this with their chirpy cheep cheeping, full of joy, waking me at 5am. Finally found a pair of old earplugs from when I used to sleep in the Snoring room and fell back asleep. Only to be woken half an hour later with the feckin sun determinedly pushing its way through the blackout blinds and curtains.

Feck it I thought – I will get up and enjoy the joys of our Summer as it is so very fleeting and may be gone by 11am. Into the bathroom and the usual cursory check in the magnifying mirror. OH MY GOD!!! The sun streams through to reveal a chin to rival Desperate Dans. A good ten minutes with tweezers follows – it's not going to be long before I have to graduate to bloody Gillette!

Then a quick shower. About to get out but then another brain fog moment – can't remember if I washed my hair while in there – so wash again just to be sure. Then the tyranny of trying on the summer clothes from the attic and realising that everything has shrunk again this year. I find a baggy maxi dress that is lovely and bright and makes me look like a hippie but will do as only alternative is to cut a hole in the duvet cover and wear it.

I find my sandals and wipe the dust off them. Bend down over my tummy (which takes some effort) to strap them up and gasp as I realise I have hairy toes!! This is some kind of sick joke by the menopause hormones – just as the hairs on my head start to thin so much that I am seriously thinking of taking my mums advice to 'have a lovely perm darling it will thicken it up – Sadie Adlington will do it for a fiver – she isn't qualified but that is just a bit of paper it will look so much better than your current flat lifeless style' – that extra hair sprouts up just about everywhere else. So deal with my toes and make a mental note (that I will instantly forget) to book a pedicure. My feet, if not my body, WILL be summer ready.

And it is only half six. I decide to treat myself to a healthy breakfast of fresh fruit and healthy juice and yoghurt in the garden. It is about a half hour walk to Tesco so I will get my exercise in and arrive just as it opens. Sweet dog agrees this is a great idea and jumps for joy. I put on my sunhat and sunglasses and look pretty cool though I say it myself.

Twenty minutes later and chub-rub has arrived with vengeance. Two naked thighs rubbing together and they are making a fire. Ouch. FFS. I remember watching something on morning telly about creating a thigh gap – it involved leaning slightly back and pushing your knees apart as if you were riding a horse. I try that and it does work though perhaps I do look a little 'special' to anyone walking past.

I get to the Supermarket determined to be healthy and regain my youthful figure. I have given up Fat Class for the Fat Lass but as I bought a pass for ten million years I still am on the Facebook page – a cursory glance this morning revealed a suggested breakfast (and this is no joke) of a Brussel sprout omelette so I think I made the right decision. I am thinking that maybe I will become a vegetarian or gluten-free or maybe lactose-free instead. Something like that. So I go a walk down the intolerant aisle and peruse the shelves. It is a little confusing so I just get chickpeas as I know for definite veggies like them and I know they make hummus which is fab for dipping my crisps into. And my fruit. And some mini chocolate ice creams because they are tiny and reduced and I convince myself I can manage to just have one a night and not the full box in one sitting. Then I realise I've forgotten a feckin bag. The mountains and mountains of feckin environmentally friendly bags at £2 each that sit behind the door and in my car ready to be used remain there as always. I cannot buy plastic bags ever since seeing Blue Planet and the Mummy Whale that would not let go of its baby that had died due to suffocating with our waste plastic. My hormones take over and I start to well up remembering it – I wave away the shop assistants look of concern. I buy another £3.50 hessian bag to add to my vast collection. I then remember I was sad the night before watching I, Daniel Blake and the lady with no money for tampons. So as I have had no period for a couple of months (could this finally be it...) I buy some 'feminine protection' to fling in the foodbank bucket. Go out to get Sweet Dog and realise I have forgotten the feckin yogurt. Back in again while – Not so – Sweet Dog goes ballistic thinking she has been abandoned. WOOF, WOOF WOOF, YOWL, YOWL – it's not a great alarm call I appreciate – but I am sure the occupants of the nearby houses would not want to waste the day by sleeping.

And finally, I head home doing my John Wayne walk to keep my thighs apart. I think of how I will lay breakfast out in the garden and how lovely it will be to sit in the sun with our healthy breakfast. I arrive back to that amazing smell of sizzling bacon. Oh my days!!! I love my partner. They are back early! Smiling above the frying pan full of lovely lovely thick smoked back bacon with a pile of white bread thick with Lurpack at the side just waiting. I put the fruit in the veg rack where it will stay 'til it goes off and fruit flies start to circulate and I tip it all in the bin – and grab the ketchup. I've had a good walk so I am due a wee treat. I can always go vegetarian another time.

Then the devil gets a hold of me – and I post a picture of my big bacon sandwich and the ice lollies on the Fat Class for a Fat Lass page just under the aubergine and sweet pea wrapped in a lettuce leaf with the simple caption 'Feck It – You only live once'.

Which is true. But if you do it right – once is enough!

NB – Brussel Sprout omelettes is not doing it right...

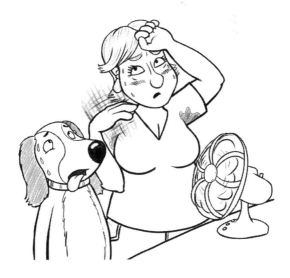

CHAPTER 16

A Room of One's Own

In this chapter I bring to you – my musings on the importance of a room of one's own to the menopausal woman.

"A woman must have money and a room of her own if she is to write fiction".

So said Virginia Woolf.

"A menopausal woman must have money and a room of her own"

So said Me!

In fact, at times I feel not just a room but perhaps a whole house or a nice sunny island. But that perhaps is a little unrealistic.

But a room – it's a start.

This is a fairly standard night for me:

10pm	Go to bed and fall asleep in six seconds flat due to being exhausted.
11pm	Wake up to go to toilet. Return to listen to snoring from partner and despair of getting back to sleep.
11.30pm	Google 'number of snorers killed by their partners.
12.00am	Get up to go to loo again. Fall asleep again.
1.30am	Nighttime Hot Flush kicks in (coz obviously 3 a day are not sufficient) – kick covers off. Partner helpfully rolls up into the kicked off quilt in sleep.
2.00am	Hot flush passes – attempt to get quilt back. Mini-argument over quilt and percentage coverage we both have of said quilt.
2.10am	Google 'menopause as a mitigating circumstance in murder of spouse'.
2.15am	Fall asleep.
3.45am	Wake up and worry about all or some of the following: getting old; lack of pension; nagging pains anywhere in body that might be a sign of a terrible illness; what might be the cause of the lump on Sweet Dogs leg.

Go downstairs to check on her. But she looks sad and lonely so worry more that lump in leg is terrible thing and give her a biscuit. Go back to bed and worry that Sweet Dog is sad and lonely. We agreed she is barred from the bed so I can't have her in with me unless my partner is away and therefore unbeknownst to them she sneaks in for a wee cuddle. I then wake my partner to check if appointment with vet tomorrow or day after. Partner not as understanding as I would like about my forgetfulness. I offer to perform a frontal lobotomy (with a rusty knife) on them so there can be full understanding of what menopausal brain fog feels like. The offer is declined.

5.30pm   Check Fitbit and worry about the lack of sleep it shows.

5.45am   Fall into a marvellous deep sleep.

6.30am   Alarm goes off for work.

This had gone on for some time – so we decide it is time for both our sanity to sleep apart. I try very hard to match my partner's disappointment while secretly (and joyously) planning the decor of MY new room and wondering how quickly the painter can come in and get it done for me.

The last time I decorated my very own room without having to consult with anyone was when I was 13 and very into Pierrot Clowns. So I got a Pierrot carpet, a Pierrot rug, a Pierrot lamp, Pierrot bedding, Pierrot curtains, Pierrot pictures, Pierrot music box, Pierrot mirror, Pierrot dolls to sit on everything; Pierrot stickers to round my window and much more – but you get the general picture. My parents were dubious but the agreement was this was it 'til I was 17 at least. At 13 I was not good at looking forward so I of course totally agreed, unable to visualise a time where I would not totally love Pierrot clowns.

That time did come – approximately 8 months later – when I became a Goth and my Pierrot clown bedroom became a total embarrassment. I was stuck with my black hair, black eyeliner and black clothes listening to moody heartbreak songs from the Cure while all around me hundreds of clowns stared disapprovingly at me.

I have learnt from that – so I clear the spare room and have it painted in nice neutral shades. I spend a large amount of money on arty prints and hide the receipts so I can pretend I got them from the charity shop for 50p each. And then last night I 'moved in'. I started in our shared bed and did the cuddly thing and had the 'yes it's for the best but so sad' conversation. We talk about Steph and Dom in Gogglebox and various other couples who have separate rooms. Finally, I judge I have spent enough time looking sad and it's time to go to my very own bedroom.

I try not to skip as I go down the hall and go into my lovely quiet beautiful room. My night goes as follows:

11.00pm: Climb into lovely clean bed.

11.30pm: Listen to Woman's Hour on Catch Up on my IPad while simultaneously doing 'snow angels' in my bed revelling in the space.

12.30am: Go to toilet. Partner shouts – 'I miss you'. 'I miss you too' I lie back.

1.30pm: Fall fast asleep.

3.00am: Wake with hot flush – simply roll to the cool side of the bed, choose one of my 'menopause playlists' from Spotify and wait for it to pass. Fall back into deep lovely sleep

5.00am: Wake up and worry for a bit. Google divorce rates in couples who sleep apart. Worry a bit more.

6.00am: Fall back asleep

6.30am: Alarm goes off – hit snooze and do some more snow angels.

We have breakfast and look at our Fitbit. I have slept about half an hour more than normal. My partner has slept an hour less and is mournful. But happy for me though because I told a bit of a white lie and said I got three hours more and feel amazing.

Because a room of one's own is a wonderful thing and I ain't giving it up.

If you too are craving a room of your own, my tip is to tell your partner that if you are rested you will be much more 'up for it' and then eat their dust as they speed to Ikea to get everything you might need for your new room.

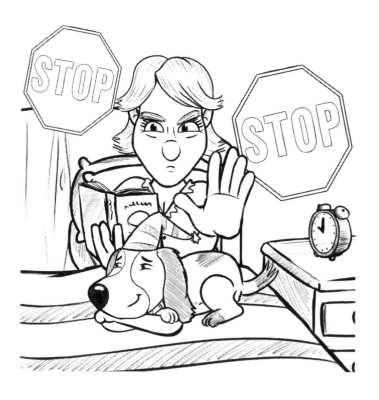

CHAPTER 17

Health Food Shop

In this chapter I bring to you – my meno-musings on my visits to the Health Food shop.

I decided a week or so again to try 'natural' help to get me through my menopause. It is a bloomin' minefield. I Googled like crazy and you could actually end up remortgaging your house if you took advice on everything. Magnesium seemed a good first choice as it claimed to reduce irritability, mood swings, insomnia and anxiety. I mean – what's not to like? So off I went to the Health Food Shop to stock up.

It was my first visit to a Health Food Shop and what an experience that was. The clientele are a bit different from Lidl that's for sure. Lots of serious-faced people with large rucksacks marching stridently up and down the lanes saying 'Excuse ME!' a lot while they compared different types of muesli that you had to scoop into a paper bag. No coco pops anywhere! I worked through seeds and nuts and tofu and oat milk and lots of similar type stuff that made me start thinking it would be a good way to lose weight – I cannot imagine sitting by the fridge eating tofu pieces out of the packet in the same way as I scoff rolled up ham with Chicken flavoured crisps in the middle. Or eating muesli at night when I come in rather than stopping off for a doner kebab. Then I discovered the sweetie section and decided that I must definitely become a vegan – at £4.20 for a bar of vegan chocolate I would be far more restrained than I am at Lidl (39p and apart from maybe some of it coming from animally things and being called 'milk chocolate', rather than some nobby title like: 'raw halo pink Himalayan salt organic coco snack', it seems to be remarkably similar). I am convinced and decide to become vegan there and then. I buy a chickpea and spinach bake which appears to resemble a Gregg's sausage roll apart from the price tag (£4.20 rather than 90p) and of course the sausage filling but how different can it really be. It will be expensive to be a vegan but it will be worth it when I am slim and healthy. I get some of the Himalayan chocolate to try on the way home.

Anyway – I have digressed. Magnesium! Supplement aisle was next. You would think it would be easy. All I want is some magnesium supplements. But nope – there are ten million types – chelated magnesium; magnesium citrate; magnesium spray – then on top of that there is a variety of strengths. I am in despair but now that I am a vegan I decide that I am in the club and can legitimately ask a member of staff. I have my chickpea bake and my vegan chocolate and a pair of vegan socks I discovered that were as soft as anything all in my basket to prove my worthiness. All the staff are about 12 and very very pale. I ask one what I should get just for a normal supplement. I pretend it is for my mum so I don't get asked any difficult questions. She hands me a bog standard magnesium supplement – success!! I leave the shop proudly displaying my eco-friendly brown health food shop making sure the logo is displayed on the outside. I am almost fifty quid down but hey ho – I am now a healthy vegan who is never going to be irritable or moody again.

Except no one told me of the bottom related side effect. I had to spend quite a bit a few days after my Health food visit in the 'little girl's room' as I played a bum symphony that would rival Beethoven's! At least I was in my own house (and I was staying there 'til I can trust my farts again!). I had the same problem at work the day before but the toilets there are not conducive to bottom explosions due to the 7 inch gap above and below the cubicle (probably summat to do with budgets – policies such as no more taxi's when you can get a bus are springing up... so perhaps no more full-size toilet cubicles is another way to save cash). This meant some serious bottom clenching when I heard people coming into toilets that were deserted when I entered. This kind of illness is a rarity for me – normally my body will not give up a calorie without some considerable fight.

I fell into a Google frenzy which will result in me convinced I have some awful disease – it can't just be an upset stomach. However, after careful deducement consisting of comparing food eaten with my partner and finding out we had eaten the same (apart from 8 Jaffa cakes and two bars of chocolate and a mint biscuit – but they have never made me ill before so I don't think it was them) and I am the only one who is ill – I conclude it is bloody magnesium supplements.

And realistically I can't spend my life on the toilet (though it would help with my aim of losing 50lbs in the 12 weeks 'til my school reunion). Apparently too much can also lead to a calcium deficiency though I am confident that my chocolate intake would always keep me out of the danger zone. But then if I am a vegan... maybe I would need to do another supplement to counteract that. I have checked other potential side effects for other supplements I was considering. Black Cohosh – weight gain and rash – so no way – Menopause has made me fat and ugly enough as it is. Ginkgo – dizziness and restlessness – can't be doing with that. Motherwort – sleepiness – well am already in bed for 9pm so that's out.

So am giving up on the supplements for now. And tbh I have to give up on the veganism as well. Well to be very honest – I gave up after an hour as the chickpea and spinach pie was absolutely awful even when I dipped it in tomato ketchup (at £4.20 I was not going to throw it away!), And also though I'd like to be slim for my college reunion – reality (and Facebook) tells me most people had also got fat – many even fatter than me.

So anyone looking for some magnesium supplements for a knockdown price (and let's face it – after reading this – how could you not?) – you can get them on my Gumtree account!

CHAPTER 18

Solo retreat

In this chapter, I bring to you – my meno-musings on taking a solo retreat.

I've been fancying a solo retreat for months. Pouring over the pictures of mountain top spas; imagining healthy tasty food served up by top-notch chefs; fantasising about long walks along a sun-kissed beach; beauty treatments that will reveal a younger more beautiful me; yoga perhaps to bring a state of stillness and calm to my monkey menopausal mind.

I saw an article with a beautiful celebrity returning from a Juicing retreat just looking so gorgeous and it inspired me to look further. SIX GRAND!! Are you kidding me?? SIX GRAND!!! My car isn't even worth that.

I check my bank balance and can just about afford £35.46.

I share my plight with a friend – and he has a great suggestion – I can have his caravan by the sea if he can use our house for the weekend. House Swap. Not quite a Portuguese coastal Health Spa but more in my price range ie free!

So off I go – alone. But not lonely. In fact, can't wait for some feckin peace! In fact, we were watching a prison drama where one of the prisoners was put in solitary confinement as a punishment and I was just thinking 'wouldn't that be bloody marvellous'. I was imagining doing a sort of Shirley Valentine but an Ayrshire Coast version rather than a Greek one. Spending my £35.46 on ready-made juices as cannot be fucked cleaning the juicer out five times a day. I also get two face masks and an intensive oil treatment for my hair from Superdrug. I find a lush bath bomb in the bathroom cabinet – a Christmas present I had forgotten about 'til now. My DIY spa is complete! I decide I will also have 2-day digital detox as I noticed one of the retreats offer that. (have a feeling they are maybe just too tight to pay for Wi-Fi).

I get to the caravan and load my stuff out, I have never been in a caravan before. Caravans are small. I am tall. I throw my bag on the bed and as I fall forward I head-butt the side of a shelf. I fall forward and clutch my head rolling on the bed in a way that would make an English footballer proud. FFS!!. I lie there in agony literally seeing stars before I get up and look cautiously in the mirror. A tiny tiny red dent. How is that possible? I feel really sick – but cannot be sick due to my body's determination to hang onto every single calorie it possibly can. I wish I had brought Sweet Dog now – she would have looked after me.

My clumsiness has certainly increased since hitting menopause. A 'funny' birthday present from my partner was a 'Mr Bump' book. How I fucking laughed!! Though I do seem particularly talented in sustaining head injuries. And am furious at whatever idiot decided to put door handles at hip height. Changes in estrogen levels cause loss of coordination and clumsiness advises my Menopause guide book. No shit Sherlock!! I so admire women who can still wear heels at this age – I can trip over my own feet in sketchers! I am quite literally an accident waiting to happen! I have been wondering about pitching the idea of a Ms Menopause book to the Mister Men franchise.

I have one of my juices and head to bed still feeling a bit sick. I am determined to have a nice 8-hour sleep. After ten mins I am wide awake – menopausal anxiety has kicked in. What if I am concussed? What if there is no mark on my head because I have internal brain damage? I feel my head – it is sore to the touch. I go back to the bathroom and examine my head in the mirror – still nothing. I debate getting my phone from the car (left there to keep out of temptation) to ask all on social media if I should head to the nearest A&E. But fall asleep before I can decide

Fortunately I wake up and am alive. I head to the bathroom and gasp in horror. There is a purple lump the size of half an egg between my eyebrows and a massive black eye is forming. I stare in morbid fascination. Fuck it – I have to get my phone and take photos and send to my nurse friends. I toddle out for my phone and the couple in the next caravan stare at me and give me a kindly smile – I smile back. 'You OK love', the husband says – 'Yes I say' – how lovely caravaners are! I try to Google concussion but there is feck all Wi-Fi.

It is odd to be alone but I carry on with my plan – five-mile hike today. I decide that a juice won't cut it so will have a full breakfast at the caravan park pub – as the pub also has Wi-Fi. The waitress in there is so kind and keeps putting her hand on my arm and asking how I am. I am attracting kindly yet pitying looks from all others. I wonder if I have dropped beans down my top. Nope. Then I go to the loo and the penny drops. I come out and I swear everyone is looking at me and it isn't just menopausal paranoia. Everyone in the caravan park thinks I am a domestic abuse victim – I am sure of it. Like Julia Roberts in Sleeping with the Enemy but fatter and spottier.

I start my hike and the wind whips up – typical after months of sun it is now a gale force wind. I struggle through then something – I think a bird – bashes across the back of my head. I scream and turn round. No-one. Nothing. I keep going and it happens again. WTF? Then I realise – it is my bloody rucksack – the clicky buttons to hold the top down aren't working so the wind is whipping it up against my head. Am getting annoyed now and resist the temptation to take it off and do a Basil Fawlty on it with one of the many sticks lying around. I do a mile more and think Fuck it – take a few selfies and lie on the beach in a sheltered corner reading my book for a bit. A completely gorgeous deserted beach. I could get used to this.

Finally get back at 5pm. And realise it was hot today. Very hot – but the bastarding wind had hidden that fact. I am burnt to bits – face, ears, and shoulders all in pain.

I want to have a cool bath with my Lush Bath Bomb but a caravan bath is about 2-foot square – so have to settle for cool shower. I am on fire!!

Next day I am more than ready to go home but decide to sit out and enjoy the sun for just a little while (keeping burnt bits covered). I realise the stones that are holding the awning bit down are hot. Very hot. And have a great idea. I pour some olive oil on them and wait for it to heat up. I rub the resulting hot oily stones on my legs (arms too burnt from yesterday) and it is heavenly. And completely free.

Last cool shower and I head for home. Looking less Amanda Holden and more like a Burns Victim that has just done 3 rounds with Mike Tyson. Not exactly the image I was aiming for.

Being alone is very good for the menopausal soul. Though being alone in a Portuguese spa for a couple of months would be even better!

CHAPTER 19

Becoming a cyclist

In this chapter, I bring to you – my musings on becoming a menopausal cyclist.

So in my ongoing fight against the symptoms of the menopause I have taken up... cycling!

Lots of reasons. As we go through the joy that is the Change (a pretty seismic change!) our body composition begins to wage war. We are all aware of the menopausal midriff that causes us to walk around as if we have an inflatable swimming tube around our middle that seems to get pumped up a bit more if we dare to as much look at a galaxy chocolate bar. But I didn't know we also start to lose lean muscle as our estrogen declines. Also, I didn't know that the changes to our body's hormones are linked to an increased risk of cardiovascular disease... and osteoporosis!

And I am still thinking of the HRT option. My patches from the menopause clinic still sit in my bathroom cupboard. According to NICE guidelines (don't know what they are called that as often they are not really very nice at all!) around 23 in every 1000 people will get breast cancer between the ages of 51–59. If you are on combined HRT that goes up by 4 – so you have a 27 in 1000 chance of getting breast cancer. However... if you are obese you have a 48 in 1000 chance. But if you take more than 2.5 hours of exercise per week then the chance drops to 16/1000.

So I am very good at hard sums and I calculated that if I do the exercise and lose the beef then go on HRT then everyone's a winner – as overall my risk level will still have dropped even if I keep taking HRT. Result!

My Exercise in Menopause guide says pick an activity you like. I had to think a lot as drinking wine in bars is something I like but they don't mean that. Also, I like eating Maltesers in front of the television. They don't mean that either. I do like trampolining but there aren't enough incontinence pads in the world to take that up. And then I remembered that joy as a kid of jumping on your bike and roaring off with pals, doing wheelies, at 8am to explore returning 'when the street lights go on' with just a few sausages wrapped in tinfoil and a packet of potato puffs (before the days of fear of predators and quinoa and kale salads for 8-year-olds).

So it was off to the bike shop. Too old to care what the 12-year-old staff think or if they take the piss behind my back – I give my requirements. Must have a MASSIVE seat – am not sawing my arse in half with those stupid ubiquitous skinny seats. Must have proper upright handlebars – as not doing a Lance Armstrong (Tour de France, not the drugs thing) and my belly would stop me leaning forward and my poor back can't take it. It must be a nice colour. I must have panniers coz not sweating with a wee rucksack on my back and need to carry water and stuff. An hour later I departed and cycled back full of joy (apart from a slight concern about how I will pay the resulting credit card bill) along the cycle path.

Which started well enough with little skippy bunnies and cherry blossom. But it would appear that most of the cycle path back to my house is littered with bad intentions! Fag packets... syringes... a ripped bed base... an old couch... group of drunk men drinking Tenants Extra and shouting 'oan yoursel – move that fat arse', as they staggered along beside me. Various bugs bite me and blind me. They also fly into my bloomin' mouth so I end up unintentionally upping my protein intake – that's karma you feckin buggy midgie things. These are things I do not recall in my childhood cycling memories!

Anyway today I decided to cycle to work. Get fit and save cash. It is only 6 miles to work – what could go wrong? My colleague kindly rocks up to accompany me. He has very smooth legs and I wonder if he maybe is a transvestite and maybe I can get an invite to one of his shows. But turns out it makes him go faster on his bike? Apparently. Suspect he may be taking the piss though he assures me he isn't. I will see how I go and maybe shave mine too – I know I need all the help I can get.

FUCK – Six Miles is a long long long long way!! A LONG WAY! After 2 miles I am sweating due to one hot flush and feckin being exhausted. Thank God there are showers in our office.

My colleague keeps charging ahead then waiting for me and I finally catch up and he tears off again 'til he is but a dot in the distance. Sometimes he turns and cycles back to get me. I should feel supported but instead tell him just to feck off and I will get there in my own time. I've also pissed myself a bit due to the bumpy road and am a bit embarrassed so I am most persuasive. So off he goes. I cannot believe how weak I feel. So I park up at the newsagent and buy a couple of chocolate bars. I think the calories burnt will make up for it.

I toddle along more sedately after this and the sugar definitely helps. I was going to have one Galaxy bar every 2 miles, but in the end I just ate them all before I left the shop and it seems to help.

I have to stop to tell my boss I will be about 60 mins late as the time estimated by my colleague turned out to be overly ambitious.

Then half a mile from the office – DUNK – the feckin seat just goes all the way down. I am sure I have whiplash and I pee myself just a little bit more. I stop and pull it up – get on and it falls back down again. Stupid thing. So I have to finish the journey with my knees hitting my chin on every turn of the pedal. Apparently you need keys by someone called Alan to fix it but the stupid bike shop didn't think to mention that.

But finally, I make it. Finally – I draw in and feel so cool and sporty just parking in the cycle bay and heading to the shower. I take my bag in and it is the best shower ever. I get out and dry off. Then go to get my work clothes. Except – except and I almost cry – there are no work clothes in my bag. None. Feckin menopausal brain fog – they are neatly piled up on my bed but not in the bag. I have no choice but to put my clean body into sweaty damp pissy disgusting leggings and t-shirt. I frantically Google trams and bikes and sigh with relief when I realise you can take bikes on the trams.

Can't possibly go to work like this – so another call to my boss to say it will be a half day for me today. Then it's up to the tram. I stop at the baker for some pain au chocolat and cycle the five mins (downhill) back to my house. Then scoff them with some hot chocolate and cream. I am fairly sure I have burned those calories off so it is fine.

I think I might need a bit more practice before I do that again. And possibly an oxygen tank. And a commitment from Lothian buses that they will keep all their buses off the roads while I am on the half-mile stretch that isn't a cycle path.

I might possibly cycle to the tram and back for a week then work up from there.

And take some sausages and potato puffs and maybe do a few wheelies.

CHAPTER 20

The Easter holidays

In this chapter, I bring to you – my meno-musings on my Easter holidays.

So – a little question for you – Guess what the Easter Bunny brought me at Easter?

A lovely big Milk Chocolate Easter Egg? Nope.

A fantastic White Chocolate Egg? Nope.

Maybe a Minty chocolate Egg? Nope

How about even just a mini one? No – wrong again!

What about an entry into a 5K? Feckin Yes! Give yourself a prize if you guessed correctly!!

Yes I swear to fecking God – a feckin entry into a 5K in May. Apparently, this is 'supportive' to my weight loss journey and will be a 'good practice' for the 10K I am doing in June which I only ended up signing up for because I was a little drunk.

OK – I did say that I didn't want an Egg due to trying to lose weight. But OBVIOUSLY I did not mean that. And if a partner of 5 years cannot see that, then I am not sure if there is a future in the relationship. And I never once mentioned or hinted that I wanted an entry into a feckin race.

I should have seen it coming – my Christmas present when we first met was 20 chickens for some African Community. I initially had to pretend to be delighted as I was portraying myself as a non-materialistic kind person (as you do at the start of a relationship). But we had a conversation over a lot of wine not long after where I explained the types of things that make good presents for me e.g. Chanel Number 5; Spa Vouchers; Posh notebooks from Paperchase; Lovely Jo Malone Candles. I don't mind having the chickens etc – but they need to be an 'extra' present – not a 'main' present. And I thought we were getting somewhere – I was having to give less and less hints to get quite good presents. Clearly we need another chat!

A feckin entry to a 5K. I mean – fuck off. I feel I may have over-reacted somewhat to the 'thoughtful gift'. But to be fair it had been a tricky few days as we were on a wee trip and as many know – the menopause can rip the 'happy' right out of holidays.

The stress had started when packing. PM (pre-menopause) it was easy – fling a few pairs of knickers in a bag with a toothbrush and some makeup and off I went.

Not now. Firstly and most importantly the tweezers have to go in. And a decision on which pair. The expensive ones that can clear a chin in 3 minutes flat or the cheaper ones that take longer but I won't mind so much if they get confiscated at Airport Security (because clearly a pair of tweezers is the weapon of choice for International Terrorists).

Then it's the menopausal supplements. My magnesium as it stops me being knackered all the time. And the chromium as it stops me eating my body weight in sugar every day.

And the medication – thyroxine because my thyroid has packed up which is common during the menopause... Dermovate because I have some odd skin condition which only flares up if I forget it... cream for my rosacea which is another lovely quite recent treat from the Menopause Fairy. Without it my face, in particular my nose, flares up making me look like a raging alcoholic.

Sanitary protection because feck knows if and when a period may appear.

Extra clothing just in case the sweats from a hot flush render an outfit no longer wearable. Extra pyjamas for the same reason.

And Sod's law – just as I need more clothes – my arse and belly increase in size and so my clothes are much bigger. Even my knickers now have to be folded before I put them in the case!

And my partner (who didn't get me an Easter egg) won't let me use their case because it is full of crap including a 2010 roadmap for when we pick up the hire car because apparently, 'satnavs are not to be trusted'. I cannot bear to once again hear the story of the car that ended up in a river when the driver followed the satnav or have another argument about how an ancient map that half the roads no longer exist on is NOT preferable to my WAZE app that will avoid traffic jams and road closures. We can have that argument later. Also – I didn't argue too much because I suspected an Easter egg might be in there... which was patently wrong!!

'Why not just pay to put an extra bag in the hold?' my partner (who didn't get me an Easter egg) said. 'Because I can think of better things to do with a 2nd mortgage' I reply. And somehow or the other I manage to cram all my stuff into my little cabin approved bag. I think we should all campaign for a free additional bag for menopausal ladies when flying. Free HRT would also be good – but failing that – the extra bag would be so useful.

And off we go – three couples ready to explore the wilds of Dorset.

But not before Airport Security. My bag whizzes through – tweezers intact – ya dancer!! But I am stopped and the lady puts the long stick thing all over me – it goes mental beeping at my fanny area. OH FECK – I forgot about my fanny magnet that reduces the desire to stab people for breathing too loud – I meant to take it off. I was most apologetic and the lady was actually quite interested so in the end we had a nice chat about it.

Tina the Turner then waltzed through setting the beeper off too. She did it on purpose though! She does it all the bloody time with her special metal bracelet – due to some fantasy she has about being frisked. I have berated her for this several times but she just shrugs and smiles as she is patted down, imaging she is in Prisoner Cell Block H or Orange is the New Black depending on her mood.

Finally we arrive at our destination airport – all sober. We pretend we are supporting the designated driver but it is really because the airline charges the GDP of a small country for a glass of wine and we forgot to pick up some vodka at the duty-free to pour into our bottles of coke.

And after ten zillion years waiting to get our hire car we all pile in and we are off. No one is allowed to look at the map apart from my partner (who didn't get me an Easter egg) and no one is allowed to use a directions app so it takes some time and a number of wrong turns and swear words to get to our final desti-nation. So the first part of my healthy eating plan for the weekend is out the window (which was to stop and get porridge for breakfast and lots of fruit and veg) as we can't be arsed going to the super-market and instead stop at an off licence then order in pizza to our cottage. I am trying to keep to the general Fat Class for the Fat Lass principles and so I start noting my 'naughty points'. Two meat-topped pizzas... Garlic bread... Ice Cream... Two bottles of wine. After that the writing gets a bit tricky to make out. I decide to give up after that – Fat Class says you should not worry if you break your diet and just start again. I suspect continually 'starting again' may be one of the reasons I am so chubby.

The next day we are all a little tender and Tina the Turner's loud and excitable nieces come to get us to take us to the 'best bar around for afternoon sessions'. We get there and my gin and tonic is served in a jam jar. A jam jar? Why would anyone want to drink their drink out of a jam jar? Apparently it is the new thing. Who knew? So I am mutton drinking as lamb. The noise is incredible and I cannot bear it. So finally us old ones feck off back to the cottage, get our pyjamas on and settle down to watch Ant and Dec – we all fell asleep halfway through it so can't say for definite.

Hot flushes, temper tantrums, fatigue and lack of an Easter egg (for the first time in nearly 50 years) aside it was a lovely holiday overall. I had lots of laughs where the tears just rolled down my legs (note to self – add incontinence pads to suitcase next time) I was feeling fairly calm and happy as we boarded the plane to come home.

But then an annoying kids TV tune came from nowhere? I looked behind me and a kid was watching their iPad in wonder. No earphones. At times like this it is hard to know if you are moody or if someone is genuinely being a twat and needs to be told. So I calmly (proud of myself) ask the mother if perhaps she has earphones for her daughter. 'Oh' she replies 'she doesn't like wearing them'. 'Oh', I reply, 'that's a shame because I doubt the rest of the plane like to listen to high pitched cartoon voices all the way home'. She compromises by turning the volume down to an annoying buzz. Does everyone get pissed off with parents who feel that playing a blaring iPad with annoying cartoons is an acceptable way to behave on public transport? Or is it just me? PUBLIC transport – the clue is in the name!

Sometimes it is nice to get home!! Peace and quiet and comfy bed. My partner who didn't get me an Easter egg offered to go and get one. But I have refused as they are half price now. I feel there may be better benefits to playing the martyr just a bit longer.

I hope you all get decent Easter Eggs from kind and thoughtful partners when Easter comes!! And if you don't they are all half price for about a week after Easter.

CHAPTER 21

A period is a pain

In this chapter, I bring to you – my meno-musings on waiting for those periods to finally go. Like a guest who has stayed around a bit too long – promising to leave but never actually going!

I was supposed to go swimming the other day. The one exercise I actually enjoy. But I am not going! Not because I am a lazy person (though tbh I am).

And not because I am barred. Though I nearly was!!! I had a nightmare swim last week when 10 zillion school kids descended on the pool meaning us adults were all corralled into two lanes and the guy behind me was so far up my arse he may as well have been my gynaecologist. I had to kick frantically to go faster and unfortunately 'accidentally' kicked him in the face.

This in itself might have been enough to get me barred as it is possible his nose may never be the same again. But he did not grass me up so I left the pool rather relieved as Google has advised me on the numerous times I have checked that the menopause is not a justifiable defence for Actual Bodily Harm in court.

I was almost barred again as I enquired at reception for the times the school children came in to use the pool. The receptionist looked appalled and asked why I wanted to know. Snotty cow I thought. But realisation dawned just before she called social services and I frantically explained I wanted to AVOID the children so I could swim in peace.

So nope – not barred. The reason I am not going is because my friend has come unexpectedly. Do you know what I mean? I have the painters in. I'm on the rag! It is star week! I have 'woman trouble'.

There are so many ways of describing your period. Germany calls it Erdeberwoche which means Strawberry Week. I particularly like Finland's description of Hallum Lechman Tauti which translates to Mad Cows Disease. This is most appropriate as I am as mad as hell. Four feckin months with nothing – NADA – and I had been lulled into a false sense of security.

I know this is normal – I know that fluctuating hormones interrupt the ovulation cycle. But this doesn't make it any easier to go back to the start of the countdown to the magical year of no periods when I can officially declare myself post-menopausal. It is a bit like when I spent 7 weeks losing half a bloody stone for my holidays through basically starving myself only to regain it all back on one all-inclusive week in Tenerife and so it was right back to the start. FFS. Some women dread this moment – a realisation that they are no longer fertile (though my pal who smugly hit 12 months with no such incidents was less smug when she discovered the last four of those months she had actually been pregnant – her baby girl is beautiful and will celebrate her 3rd birthday at the same time as my friend celebrates her 50th, Turns out fertility does not disappear neatly with the onset of perimenopause as she had originally thought. Her 16 & 18-year-olds are great babysitters though) But I cannot feckin wait to be shot of my periods. No more spending money on sanitary products instead of gin. No more paying VAT because someone somewhere declared them a luxury. No more wondering when it will appear from nowhere (usually when wearing very pale trousers). Bring it on.

Except my body keeps playing tricks on me. Months pass with nothing and I think I am almost there. Then Mother Nature sends her guest down and pisses herself laughing at my distress. Especially today – when I have my best knickers on (£8.99 from Autograph!).

And of course, I have nothing with me – no sanitary protection at all. Good news though – our forward-thinking employer has installed a machine in the toilet where for 50p I can have a nice sanitary towel.

I wrestle with the machine and finally manage to get one of the most massive bulky towels I have ever seen out of a very tiny tray. But needs must. I think of Alanis Morrisette's song 'It's like ten thousand knives when all you need is a spoon'. Well, this is like ten thousand pads when all I want is a tampon. Though it is possible my fanny might have closed up due to lack of action – with my current bedroom fantasy is watching catch up telly while eating chocolate. I had a scone once but the crumbs went everywhere so it was straight back to dependable chocolate.

The bloomin' pad is huge – and has no wings to keep it in place. I walk gingerly around with this monstrosity balancing in my lovely knickers with the lace edges that are not designed to keep towels safely locked in. For the first time, I am glad to have pudgey thighs rather than a thigh gap coz there is less chance of it falling out. I don't get embarrassed easily now. I used to – in second-year at school Mark Nimmo saw a tampon in my school bag and took it out and threw it across the classroom, I thought I would have to leave school and never return, such was my mortification. But over the years I have been significantly more embarrassed by a number of events and so nowadays very little embarrasses me – but even I might be somewhat abashed if I am queueing up at the canteen for a galaxy and the towel was to fall down my trouser leg onto the floor!

I remember the days I looked forward to my period coming – proof that all was in working order and I was most definitely not pregnant. Now I look forward to that magical 1 year period free when I will never see it again!

CHAPTER 22

A rant about International Women's Day

In this chapter, I bring to you – a meno-rant about International Women's Day (or at least how some men choose to interpret it)

I really wish this was an inspirational musing to celebrate International Women's Day.

But it isn't. Coz I am raging. And that makes me rant.

So I am going to have to give in to it I'm afraid.

I got to work on International Women's Day last year – and my colleague Jane told me that all the women in our team have been sent a lovely email for Women's Day from one of the men in another team.

I open it up – there is an image of a bunch of flowers and a message saying 'International Women's Day – a day for us men to thank all you girls for being so nice and adorable and doing all the hard work to give us our beautiful children'

"Isn't that lovely?" Jane said

"Are you fecking kidding me?" I responded. "Is he fecking serious?"

Jane has heard a lot of my rants over the last year or so – and obviously wanted to escape so she quickly started taking coffee orders while I simmered away glaring at the email trying to think of a suitable response.

Turns out he had a number of less than complimentary responses (which gives me hope) and is all upset as he doesn't know what he has done wrong – another email arrives from him apologising for causing any offence but that he 'genuinely wanted to extend his thanks and does not understand why everyone is annoyed'.

Aww diddums...

I drink the lovely latte that I am brought and nibble on the accompanying chocolate bar (which I think she only bought me to stop me talking for a while) and come up with my response:

Hello A. Ness (his parents named him Andrew Ness not realising he would spend the rest of his life being called Anus).

1. *You have kind of missed the point – International Women's Day is a worldwide event that celebrates women's achievements – from the political to the social – while calling for gender equality. It is not a day for men to thank women for being 'nice'. In fact – strange thought it may be to comprehend – the day is not about men at all.*

2. *Yes – we are women – none of us are under 25 therefore we are most definitely not girls.*

3. *I have no kids – this does not make me less of a woman than someone who does.*

4. *I am not 'nice' or 'adorable' – and again this does not make me any less of a woman who is.*

Regards

I deliberately don't put 'Kind Regards' as I normally would so he can see just how pissed off I am.

He comes over to join us at lunchtime, clearly anxious that our (admittedly overzealous) HR team may find out about all of this and send him on the dreaded Diversity course. I wasn't really ready to play nice on account of still being as mad as hell – so decided to instigate chat around what we can do to improve women's rights which he has to talk about as he is trying hard to get into our good books again.

Out of ten of us – only 2 agreed with quotas to improve the number of women in board positions. ONLY 2. I was one – and in real rant mood so took over most of the conversation.

I absolutely believe in quotas – I have seen too many boardrooms in different organisations made up TOTALLY of white middle-class men. Don't try to tell me that for every single one of those posts there wasn't a single woman out there that could have done that role. I am so over having doubts about this kind of thing.

Someone was brave enough to comment that if women were given posts just because they are women then we'd end up with rubbish women in the jobs. I get a bit irked again. I beg to feckin differ. Firstly because this implies that there are no decent women available for these jobs. Also – for decades (centuries even) men have been given posts just because they are men and we end up with some rubbish men in some jobs. So why can't we have a few rubbish women, just because they are women, to balance it up?" I get a bit worked up here and talk quite fast and I know some people are thinking I am mad but I know what I mean. It is bloody ironic that just as I get to the age of being confident enough to vocalise my opinion that brain fog kicks in to make me less eloquent than I was when I was younger and was too scared to say what I thought.

Anyway, most people avoided me for the rest of the day because they know that a rant can now last all day. I think they were relieved when I decided to head for home a bit early

I stopped at the newsagent and I had to have another rant to myself when I saw all the covers of the papers. Pictures of one or the other of the Kardashians, Cheryl Whatever She is Called Nowadays, Kerry and her 5000 kids and her boobs hanging out all over the place... story after story about fat women becoming thin, thin women becoming fat... women getting plastic surgery etc. Nothing at all against them but where are the other woman who are truly inspirational?

I can bet if you pulled 50 people off the street and ask if they knew who Cheryl/Kim Kardashian/Kerry Katona are – they would all know.

But what about Cressida Dick? Mary Barbour? Victoria Drummond? Marie Stopes? Rosa Parks? Malala Yousafzai? Benazir Bhutto? Gloria Steinem? Amelia Earhart? Shami Chakrabarti? Anita Roddick? Florence Price? Joan of Arc? Mhairi Black? Nicola Sturgeon? Angela Merkal? Are they inferior just because they don't/didn't go to work in their underwear? Because they didn't break the internet by pouring champagne over their shoulder onto their bum or whatever it was? (I am mad that I even know this...)

Take Mary Barbour first. After WW1 started, 1000s of workers flocked to Glasgow for work in the shipyards and munitions factories. Greedy property owners tried to profit by pushing rents up through the roof. Mary wasn't for it and worked to mobilise working-class families, especially women, to challenge the power of landlords and organise a rent strike. Her actions led to the passing of one of Europe's first Rent Restriction Acts. She didn't stop there though – campaigning for better homes and finally becoming the first fully fledged woman magistrate of the city of Glasgow. She was also of the leading movers in Glasgow's first Birth Control clinic.

Victoria Drummond – received an MBE for bravery at sea during WW2 when she single-handedly kept the engines of the SS Bonita running while under German bombardment.

Benazir Bhutto – the first female prime minister of a Muslim Country – moving Pakistan from dictatorship to democracy and bring in social reforms to help women and the poor.

I could go on... But the point is they did so much to pave the way for us. And yet awareness of them is low compared to the celebs of today who see activism as clicking like on a Facebook post about a march... or who see typing hashtags with their favourite cause as a major contribution to its success...

Trying to be positive – we have obviously made huge strides in the last few years thanks to the women who fought for the rights we have today. But I can't help feeling there is some way to go.

Happy Women's Day to all the Fabulous Women out there.

CHAPTER 23

Fat Class for the Fat Lass, the sequel

In this chapter I bring to you, my musings going back to Fat Class for the Fat Lass after being on a 'break'.

Two and a half pounds ON!!! I kind of knew it coz I did stick to the plan but over and above it I had 6 bottles of wine, four meals out, three fry ups (not done in spray oil), four bars of chocolate, six Jack Daniels and coke, a kebab and a fish supper. But I was on holiday!! I gave up counting the 'naughty points' after the first fry up as even though I am good at sums I just couldn't be arsed – I was in the holiday mood. Two of my holiday companions were also fatter than me so I just made sure I stood beside them for photos. Also when I am a bit drunk I don't really care about being fat anymore and I was a bit drunk for a lot of the holidays.

So it was all fun and games 'til I saw the photos on Facebook and had to spend quite some time messaging various people to get them to delete them and NEVER EVER to post a photo of me looking a size 20 again. And yes I KNOW I AM a size 20 but for God's sake – Photoshop!

So I decided to go back to Fat Class as I had a 12-week pass and am not wasting it. But not to hang about in class – just do the walk of fat shame from the scales to the door and run for it. I was not the only one. We all had our excuses at the ready – some more plausible than others. One of the members declared that she knew she had gained this week as she just 'hadn't eaten enough'. I love her optimism!! Yep – another six chocolate bars and you would have nailed it!!

Another felt she had just not drunk enough water and that is why she gained 5lbs. And another had walked to work twice that week and had read that 'muscle weighs more than fat' and that was the reason for her 2lb weight gain. I was a little confused – surely a lb of muscle weights the same as a lb of fat? And also I can see the athletes at the Commonwealth Games using that as a valid excuse but not someone who had done 2 x 20-minute walk in a week.

Another said in a quiet whisper it was her 'star week'. One of the guys was most confused but regretted asking when he got a detailed explanation of her menstrual cycle. The Leader was most understanding and made a wee note beside her name. Another four weeks 'til she can use that excuse again!

I also couldn't cope with more happy-clappy stuff. So I decided to use the time to do something more productive – a trip to the supermarket as I have laid out our menu for the entire week to get back on plan. And it is a very long list full of ingredients that would not normally go into my basket so we may be there some time!

I had looked at our Fat Class for the Fat Lass private Facebook page for inspiration on recipes. Me and my partner invented an interesting game of 'do you know what it is yet?' using the pictures on the page – you are welcome to steal this game – it passes things like 2-hour delays in airports! My partner guessed the first one to be deep fried dog turd on radioactive nuclear waste. That was wrong – it was actually Fat Lass Meatballs on Broccoli Rice. But we gave half a point because to be fair it did look like something you would use a poop scoop on.

The page may achieve its aim of ensuring its reader's weight loss though – as after reading it I was so nauseous I did not want to eat for a good half hour. I have saved some of the pictures on my phone so I can look at them if I want to stop myself eating. I mean – really – a cabbage and leek omelette? I would not want to be downwind of the diner of that particular dish a few hours later!!

We did wonder if someone was talking the piss – one proud wife showed the dinner her husband had ready for her – a baked potato with a grilled courgette, fried mushrooms, ten crabsticks and a tin of beans on top!!! She declared him a 'keeper'!

Another posted their breakfast – five fried eggs, ten rashers of bacon, mound of fried mushrooms, and six SW sausages. 'All unlimited food' the caption boasted. Hmm – I like an avocado chopped up on my toast sometimes but avocado BAD according to Fat Class. Very BAD – so full of naughty points that I would have to say several Hail Mary's if I gave in to temptation!! But hey a heart attack on a plate is absolutely fine.

We decided to use a modicum of common sense. So we had a doughnut to take away the 'taste' of those images and planned out some meals using our Fat Lass app. We wrote them all up on our white board and were most impressed and had a good laugh as we looked forward to our slim summer bodies.

We were not laughing an hour later in Tesco. 'Do we actually need feckin Quark?' my partner asked after a frustrating search down several aisles of yoghurts and creams. 'YES' I said – we need it to make our curries smoother and our pasta dishes less dry and to put on meringues to make them delicious for just one tiny naughty point. It is the answer to EVERYTHING! Perhaps even world peace! We need them to cook every bloody thing for the full feckin week – KEEP LOOKING!!' Finally I Googled it – feckin soft cheese! Who would put soft bloody cheese on a meringue? We bought several pots as it IS mission critical for Fat Lass success. And my partner will do anything that even just possibly eases the menopausal symptoms that have blighted me over the last few months. (Not enough Hail Marys in the world to atone for some of the things I have done and said... oops... some were on purpose tbh but I just blamed the menopause anyway).

Another half hour of arguments and trailing up and down aisle after aisle debating such things as would mixed herbs would be a good replacement for the myriad of expensive spices required? Would we need a second mortgage to buy all this stuff? But no – if we are doing it we are doing it right so we bought every last thing on the list. But we were quite knackered then and I remembered two things – the sharpie pens that the lady at fat class brought in so we could 'draw a line' under our naughty few days and also the concept of 'flexing those naughty points' where if you feel like it you just eat what you want and start again the next day. So as we passed the reduced aisle we spotted a curry meal for four down to a tenner so we got that and some onion bhajis and some of those cream doughnuts with the strawberry sauce on them. And a bottle of white. But we are DEFINITELY drawing a line under this and starting properly tomorrow.

We almost fainted at the checkout when it came to £210 instead of our usual £40 but we reassured ourselves that most of this was stuff for our 'cupboard essentials' which up 'til now consisted of Pringles, Squashies and chocolate eclairs. But now we are doing things RIGHT. No more grabbing a square sausage and potato scone roll in the work canteen in the morning – NO Siree – we will be taking our fruit and yoghurt in. No more fish and chips for lunch – we will have our salmon and salad and fruit. No more meals out – we will be going a brisk walk then back for a tasty king prawn curry made with lovely creamy Quark.

Note to Fat Class for the Fat Lass – a spoon of Quark on a meringue is NOT an acceptable replacement for double cream... just saying!

CHAPTER 24

Just another fucker of a day

In this chapter I bring to you – my meno-musings on my visits on days that can only be described as fuckers.

The term 'fucker of a day' was coined by someone who had a day just like the one I had a few weeks ago

It was the last day of work before some annual leave – I head off to Glasgow and am almost there before I remember today is a day for the Edinburgh office and have to do a fecker of a reroute back (they should put bloody bridges a mile or so after every slip road so if you miss it you can just come back!) It should be law that forgetful menopausal women can only work in one place!

Also, none of my colleagues seem to have got the memo that on the last day before your holiday you do very little apart from turn on your 'out of office' and give everyone a regular countdown throughout the day of how long it is before you start your holidays. No – my colleagues got some other memo that said irritate the fuck out anyone going on holiday by asking them to meetings to discuss how things can stay 'on piste' in their absence or how x project can 'maintain its flightpath'. And I had to pretend to be interested in all the things that would happen while I was lying on a beach drinking cocktails.

Finally I got to bugger off home and would have loved to have gone on a pre-holiday spa – get my nails and hair done etc particularly the toenails due to menopausal midriff tendering the necessary bending a huge challenge. But I am suffering from 'menopausal poverty' which is the fresh hell you get after years of 'period poverty'. Having to spend money on things like magnesium supplements; Incontinence pads; a bigger size of clothes every two months; new shoes to cheer yourself up; buying friends lunch to make up for calling their husbands tossers when in the midst of 'menopausal honesty moments'; new glasses as your sight decides to give up the ghost as well as various other parts of your body; waxing and laser treatment for all the excess facial hair; dying the grey from your hair; getting the odd weird skin tag thing removed; slimming club memberships all adds up.

There should be a tax allowance for menopausal women!!

But the government is too busy stealing our pensions to think of that so instead of a lovely £400 spa I decide to have a relaxing bath with magnesium flakes in it (£3.95 for a pouchful – Holland and Barret); a large glass of red wine (£4.99 a bottle Aldi); and a mint club (£1 for a pack of 5 in Asda) while wearing a special face mask (99p Superdrug) thus saving £390.95. I mean it's not exactly Champneys but it will do.

And it was quite nice 'til Sweet Dog decided to try and get in the bath with me for some reason that I will probably never fathom. In pushing her out I spilt my red wine and my mint club fell in the water. But there is no way I was getting out of that bath as the magnesium flakes were expensive and the instructions insist you stay submerged for 20 mins for maximum benefit!

My partner comes in and screams. And I nearly jump out of my skin as I was just dozing off. 'What the fuck is wrong with you? I am trying to relax' I shout. But I kind of see where 'the fear' may have come from – I am lying with a mask that makes me resemble Hannibal Lecter in a bath that looks like it is blood with what they thought was a large poo floating beside me (not realising it was a melting mint club).

I am a little disappointed as the HRT is boosting my libido but I suspect this isn't the best foreplay and my luck may not be in!

Anyway – they have bought the dinner so I am a little bit happier. I decide to check Facebook while they cook it. It greets me with a premenopausal photo from 8 years ago looking young fresh-faced and not the kind of person that considers stabbing people on a regular basis. I wonder if I can disable the 'memories' – I mean they are not often happy – eg. oh look here is your dead granny from 10 years ago'/'oh remember your dog you adored that is now dead? No? You had just got over it? Ha Ha – here is a picture to rub it in'... etc...

And I check the fridge and am even more raging. Can I ask – who on this planet gets cheese as a desert? I mean really? The cheese? I know for a fact there was a profiterole stack and millionaire chocolate dessert as options in the meal deal options. WHO PICKS THE BLOODY CHEESE OVER THAT? It is times like this that I wonder if we are suited at all and maybe we should just end it due to 'irreconcilable differences' in what constitutes a good pudding.

But then I remember the other four mint clubs!! So not a complete total fucker of a day! And it is holiday time tomorrow. No more working for a week or two. We are going where the sun better feckin shine brightly and the sky better be feckin blue (to paraphrase Cliff Richard!).

CHAPTER 25

To HRT or not to HRT

In this chapter, I bring to you – my meno-musings on: to HRT or not to HRT.

Because I'd been asking myself this question for some time.

As that is the question I have been asking myself for a few months since I was given a prescription but was too afraid to start it.

As mentioned before, I have pored over the evidence. Not in the way a medical scientist would maybe recognise as research – as it is mainly checking what celebrities have been on HRT then watching programmes like Loose Women and This Morning carefully to see the effects.

It was in 1966 that HRT started to come to prominence with Dr Wilson, in his book 'Forever Feminine' describing the menopause very much as a disease that could be treated. He advocated HRT as a way to keep your husband happy. My Menopausal Monster hackles rose reading this – and tbh reading many articles written even in the last year or two which seem to think that the driving force for all women seeking help is to ensure their husband/partner can get a good shag. Indeed I have yet to read anything that says if you can't be arsed (due to sweating your tits off, being utterly exhausted and worrying about the possible consequences of telling a work colleague this morning to feck off) then you should just say you can't be arsed, go to bed and tell your partner to bring you some wine, a bar of galaxy and a cool compress then feck off to the spare room so you can watch Netflix in peace.

In fact how about one of those Gadgety Mags that men read having a wee article on how to look after a menopausal woman. And they maybe explain that when a menopausal woman is lying in bed and suddenly rips off all her clothes it is unlikely that his luck is in and instead of leaping on top of her, he should open a window, bring out a large fan then go and get some chocolate for her.

Anyway back to the point – it turned out his book was funded by one of the biggest manufacturers of HRT – which pissed me off even more than the content of the book. Though my bra was also really pissing me off that morning – so it doesn't take much.

I have played about with fanny magnets and magnesium but tbh I have pretty much been self-medicating with rum, white wine and Family Sized chocolate bars. And I have to concede that this does not seem to be helping my 'disease'. So maybe it is time to try something else.

I expand my research outwith the confines of OK and Closer – but end up more confused than ever.

'Go on it' advocates say. 'Your risk of osteoporosis and colon cancer will reduce. Your insomnia and hot flushes will go. You will be a sparkly happy sexual being again'.

'Don't go on it' say the detractors. 'You may end up with endometrial cancer, gallbladder problems, breast cancer and dementia'.

I mean – talk about a rock and a hard place.

I am not sure how I feel about pumping my body full of unnatural hormones. And I suppose if I am honest – it feels like a 'failure' to start taking them – after all, isn't this just another phase of life?

I told that to my friend Clare Obama, and she asked me if I could remember what I told her when I visited her after she had her first baby. I can't actually remember what I had for my breakfast – so I had to admit that a memory from 20 odd years ago would be quite tricky.

She reminded me that she had been devastated as she had to have a C-Section and had cried her eyes out to me explaining she felt like a failure for not having a natural birth.

I am still looking blank and panicking slightly that I have no recollection of this.

'You said you begged to feckin differ and then called me a fuckwit and told me I cooked a gorgeous baby girl and who gave a shit if she came out my fanny or belly button or even got delivered by a bloody stork'

I still don't remember.

'You also brought two fantastic chocolate eclairs'. I have a glimmer of recall now – I do remember them. They were fantastic.

So she calls me a fuckwit and tells me that no one gives a shit if I take something that isn't natural. She also reminded me that it was synthetic cream in the eclairs coz neither of us liked 'natural' cream.

So I decided I was doing it – HRT for me. I want to be gorgeous like Andrea McLean and springy and jumpy like Davina and have a big smile like Lorraine. And I have a pal that claims her marriage and job and sanity were all saved by HRT which made her feel herself again. And if HRT can make me feel like me again – then

I don't care if it isn't natural. I miss me a lot. (though Google says that some HRT has the Urine of Pregnant Horses in it – and that seems fairly natural).

So off to the Doctors I go, happy that I have made a decision.

But five minutes later I change my mind. I absolutely don't want to use them. But when I arrive – I am absolutely sure that I do. Then ten minutes later I am not sure again. Then I decide absolutely not.

The Doctor tries to give me anti-depressants which I thought might be nice. But then I am sure I am not depressed. I think. I just am not sure.

I am sure of wanting cake though so on the way home I nip into the baker's for two massive Chocolate Eclairs filled with synthetic cream. I try to give the impression that one is for me and the other is for someone who has just had a baby – but I know she knows that I know that one is for now and the other is for when I get home to have with a cup of tea.

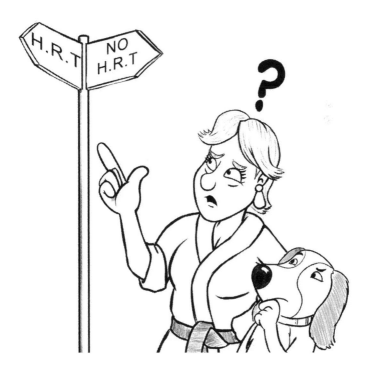

CHAPTER 26

Family Support

In this chapter I bring to you, my meno-musings on the support a menopausal woman can get from their family

It was a ladies lunch with aunties and the mothership and cousins when I decide to ask my older female relatives their experience of the perimenopause and menopause. (my menopause book says I should ask as I am likely to go through a similar process).

Within twenty mins I am thoroughly depressed (my younger cousins are wearing similar depressed expressions but taking comfort in the possibility that a cure will be found by the time they get there) as it would appear all the older female members of my family had long drawn out awful menopauses where they were lucky to avoid jail/being sectioned/being on social services radar. My mum insists hers lasted 25 years – I panic and Google it on my phone secretly under the table and am relieved to find that 8 years seems to be the maximum. I'd rather trust Google than my mum. Her medical expertise is limited – she insists to any overdue expectant mother that they should refuse to be induced as the baby will come in its own time – and adds I was due at the start of August and arrived in my own good time in the middle of October. (I was 6lbs 13oz – I don't need Google to know her theory is highly unlikely). "Auld age doesn't come by itself" she muses.

Then Auntie Michelle who has been fairly quiet suddenly declares that the menopause is just like puberty and women just need to accept that and know that it will pass and get on with it.

"Just like puberty? Seriously?' I say.

"Yes," she says – "look at puberty as the opening bracket of the reproductive and sexual part of your life and the menopause as the closing bracket"

That doesn't really cheer me up. It is also embarrassing as my aunt is a bit deaf and therefore shouts rather than talks and we are in a restaurant. Several people turn as the word 'sexual' was bellowed out. Heads shake as the word 'menopause' was bellowed out twice.

"Remember you moped about all the time, snapping at everyone who asked you how you were" she continued. "And you just listen to a tape of that Cure band all the time and dyed your hair jet black – and you had that massive crush on Christine Cagney. Well, it's the same now – except its Helen Mirren you have a crush on. And you dye your hair blonde now. Yes – it's like you are 14 all over again" she repeats, laughing merrily away.

Oh yes – it's exactly like I was 14 again! Exactly like it – apart from:

- Occasionally peeing myself whenever I sneeze or laugh too much.

- Being five stone heavier with the weight I used to put on my legs and boobs now pooling around my tummy (though one benefit is I can rest my dinner plate on it now).

- Needing tweezers not just for my eyebrows but for various other random parts of my face.

- Worrying about everything rather than just how to nick a blue eyeshadow from Woollies and whether dewberry or white musk perfume from the Body Shop would be best for the School Disco.

- Not having regular 'whooshes' of excitement for the future and what it might hold because according to my menopause book it is likely to hold osteoporosis, cardiovascular disease, thinning hair, zilch sex life and depression. Whoop de feckin whoop!!

- Regularly feeling like I have an internal radiator that ramps up whenever I least expect or want it.

- Having sagging skin and wrinkles rather than smooth silky even skin (I wish I had appreciated that more!!)

- Waking up at least three times a night to visit the loo.

Menopause is just like puberty? I beg to feckin differ. And actually – my hair is blonde – I just have a few highlights put in to brighten it up. And it wasn't 'the Cure band'. It was just 'The Cure'. And they were cool. I actually preferred Alison Moyet and Yazz and the Communards. But it was cool to like the Cure. And I wanted to be cool.

That is one good thing I suppose – as well as giving very few fucks about anything, I don't feel any need to be cool any more. That is quite liberating. I know I should proclaim to like London Grammar and other cool bands for 40 something people – but I quite like One Direction and I think Justin Bieber does some good songs too. And Jesse J does some songs to make you think too. And

Helen Mirren is a goddess and a national treasure and therefore it is fine to have a girl crush on her too.

I just remembered that Christine went through the menopause on Cagney and Lacey!!! I didn't really understand it at the time – but it was an episode towards the end – she had hot flushes. I spend a happy rest of the day with chocolate watching old episodes.

CHAPTER 27

My ever-changing moods

In this chapter, I bring to you – my meno-musings on my ever-changing moods

- Pre-menopause, my moods could be roughly categorised thus:
- Happy for a reason – 50% of the time
- Happy for no particular reason – 10% of the time
- Grumpy for a reason – 20% of the time
- Grumpy for no reason – 10% of the time
- Tearful for a reason – 5% of the time
- Tearful for no reason – 5% of the time.

Things have changed somewhat – since the menopause the categories are thus:

- Happy for a reason – 10% of the time
- Happy for no particular reason – 5% of the time
- Grumpy for a reason – 10% of the time
- Grumpy for no reason – 50% of the time
- Tearful for a reason – 1% of the time
- Tearful for no reason – 24% of the time.

And as I am still having periods, PMT also arrives at random points to join the menopausal party in my head.

This can lead to so many emotions in one day. One minute I am in tears watching an advert with a lonely man with no friends in it and reaching for my phone to donate my week's salary to help him go to a wee club on a Tuesday afternoon. The next I can be as mad as hell about my partner putting the paper in the wrong recycling box. Or walking out of the Supermarket in a rage because once again they have changed the layout of the store and I can't find the feckin milk!

The other day, the menopause and the PMT combination was at a height – I was happy in the morning. I was heading out in my lovely new car to do some shopping with some Christmas vouchers. All was well in the world and I sang along cheerily to the radio.

I then got to the multi storey car park which seems to have shrunk since I bought my bigger car. I started a bit of grumpiness – justified I think because the spaces are just too bastarding small. Then I was completing a particularly complex parking manoeuvre and struggling somewhat. So I was getting even grumpier. Again – I think quite justified.

Then I saw in the rear view mirror a 'wide boy' in the car behind – gesticulating and, although I don't do sign language, the movements of his mouth hinted at language that wasn't particularly compli-mentary. So I get really really grumpy. And then I thought – fuck it – I am too old for some wee shit to try and intimidate me. I get out the car – with grumpiness now off the scale and approach his car. He rolls the window down and looks at me blankly but I detect a little fear which gives me great satisfaction.

"What. The. Fuck. Is. Your. Problem?" I roar.

He looks blankly at me again – and I start to get an inkling something isn't quite as I assumed. Then a disembodied female voice fills the car 'are you alright babe?' Feck... Feck... Feck...

He was talking on his hands-free to his girlfriend. He wasn't being a shit – just talking while he waited. 'I'm sorry' I say – 'I thought you were shouting at me'. I start to feel very tearful.

'I'll call you back babe' he says to his girlfriend. He then says – 'Are you OK? I'm sorry – I didn't mean to upset you, I was just talking to my girlfriend', He is gentle and kind and I suspect he works in mental health or something similar where he has gained a lot of practice in dealing calmly with unreasonable angry women. So then I was sobbing at his loveliness and thinking what a good job his parents have done.

After this debacle, I Google paranoia as a symptom of the menopause. And yes – it is another sweet symptom. Apparently if I go for a walk it will help! I beg to feckin differ. I walk Sweet Dog for miles and it isn't helping at all.

I have reflected a bit on the sudden rages and irritability that currently blight my life. Apparently it is all the fluctuating hormones that cause my rollercoaster of emotions. Dropping levels of estrogen are associated with low levels of serotonin (the 'feel good' hormone). Thought, to be honest, I can't blame the menopause completely – since a very young age I have felt a desire to hit certain people over the head with a sharp object. But taking the positive from this – I now have nearly 50 years' experience of not giving in to my impulses. The problem is that these impulses are now combined with the lack of fucks given at this time of life which makes me – well it makes me a piece of glass hidden in the sand ready to cut when you least expect it. And Helen Mirren hasn't really helped by saying that if she could give her younger self some advice then she would tell her to tell others to fuck off more often. I respect Helen Mirren and subconsciously I think I am taking on board her advice.

A couple of weeks ago I was on a bus – and some arse was drinking from his can of Tenants and singing some rude football chant and trying hard to engage his rather embarrassed girlfriend to join in.

Seeing my face, he slurred 'giesasmiledoll' (this is a language known in Glasgow as 'Bampot' – the English translation is: 'Please can you cheer up and smile at me')

So I did what most British people would do and stared at my phone as if some very important message had just come through and I must read it very carefully.

He was not to be put off. '"Umahaffendinyamissus' (again this is bam pot language, the translation is: "Am I offending you?')

Helen Mirren's advice popped into my head and I tried to ignore it.

Suddenly I heard someone say 'Aye you are offending me – so why don't you take your tiny shrivelled dick and get off the fucking bus at the next stop and give us all some fucking peace'

It took a moment before I realised that it was actually me that had said that. The filter between my brain and my mouth seems to have developed a severe fault.

The bus took a collective gasp – then... and only in Glasgow would this happen... I got a wee round of applause.

I couldn't help myself. 'You' I said, pointing at the girlfriend 'can do better than THAT' and pointed at the Arse (whose face was now slack in disbelief).

I got off at the next stop to a round of cheers from the bus (my actual stop was another three on but I was getting a little scared of the angry drunk man who looked like he was planning cruel and unusual revenge).

I am not sure if it was good, bad or stupid... But it felt quite good.

I check Google to see if Menopause is every used as a mitigating circumstance in a criminal court. It doesn't appear so. So I have decided to start sorting these ever-changing moods out.

My fanny magnet does seem to help... though clearly given evidence above it hasn't completely stabilised my emotions. I have had a look at the various supplements recommended but it is a bloody minefield. And I really don't want another trip to the Health Food Shop. Some sites say there is no scientific evidence to back up their effectiveness. Others say they will make you as serene as Jane Seymour. There are also so many of them – magnesium, chromium, vitamin B12; vitamin B6; Black Cohosh and a million others. But will they help? They are so bloomin' expensive. But maybe I will do some more research. I might have a wee look and see what is available online. And then I am just going to pick one. Just one. For the moods.

I just checked Google again – if you are suffering the same – you are in good company. 70% of menopausal woman describe irritability as the main emotional problem of the menopause.

Maybe as a tribute to the lovely poet Jenny Joseph who died not that long ago we should all "make up for the sobriety of our youth" and give ourselves permission to do exactly as we please now and then (unless that involves being horrible lovely young man who's driving a red Corsa and probably works in mental health – just be lovely to him if you see him).

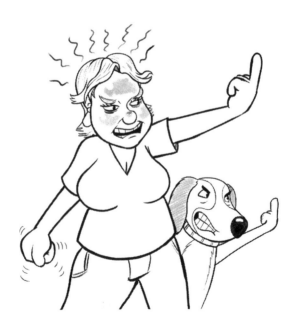

CHAPTER 28

Going Vegan

In this chapter, I bring to you – my menopausal musings on Going Vegan.

The first 9 hours I was vegan went really well.

I have been thinking about it for a while and have been reading up on it. Apparently all animals are given hormones to speed up their growth. And if they are eating hormones – then you are also eating their hormones when you eat meat. And as the balance of my hormones at the moment is decidedly precarious then this is perhaps a complication best avoided.

It is also claimed that eating soy and soy foods regularly can help alleviate menopausal symptoms because it contains something called phytoestrogens which reduce hot flushes. Even better some research says that soy can fight the diseases the Menopause Fairy likes to bring along such as high cholesterol, osteoporosis and heart disease.

However, the deciding factor was watching Carnage while recovering from a hangover this morning. Me and my pal sat with piles of chocolate and found it on iPlayer. We thought it would be funny coz Simon Amstell produced it. Well, it wasn't. Nothing has ever put me off Galaxy but when I saw the horrible man drag the crying calf away from its mummy so they could steal all the baby's milk from its devastated mother to make chocolate bars I could not eat it anymore – I swear I could taste the despair. And just when I thought my menopausal moods were starting to stabilise, I spent some time alternating between crying my eyes out and feeling fury.

So it was off to the book shop to get some vegan cookbooks and then on line to order all my vegan supplies. Then a quick trip to Lakeland to get a waffle maker for the sweet potato waffles and a Tofu press.

I returned home to find my partner less than supportive – especially when I lift all Lakeland bags out of the boot. "NOOOHHHHHH" was the response "You promised you would not go into Lakeland for at least a year when we worked out that we had £1400 worth of their products in the attic gathering dust"

"We are going vegan" I replied calmly. "It is a new way of living. If you want to eat meat and eggs that is fine but don't expect me to cook it for you"

"I do most of the bloody cooking coz you always say that you are menopausally exhausted and can't be arsed – so how exactly will that work" is the next response which is also less than helpful.

"Not a feckin problem," I say. "I will go for my tea at Wagamamas every night if that is how you feel and you can just stuff yourself full of dead cows yourself. So it is ABSOLUTELY FINE". But all women know that 'absolutely fine' does not mean fine – it means 'I am in a huff and you won't be getting any for quite some time!'

"What about bacon sandwiches on a Sunday?" my partner says sensing a weak spot.

But I have thought of that. I do like a crispy bacon sandwich and even watching Babe didn't stop me eating bacon. "That's ok" I reply – "I will have them still – but for the rest of the week I am going to be completely vegan"

'Right... so you are going to be a vegan who eats bacon sandwiches on a Sunday... just so I am sure?" is the next response as my partner ponders my logic.

I don't answer for a minute as I am looking at the Fat Gay Vegan website on my phone. But the silence is getting a bit deafening so I have to clarify. "I am not going to be a wankyvegan that thinks courgette and beetroot traybake is a good alternative to chocolate fudge cake – and makes a big fuss in restaurants to get attention. But I am serious – apart from that I will be totally vegan."

"Oh for fuck's sake" is the response "It is a bloody fad – like that time you went all Deliciously Ella and spent £400 on a Magimix because she insisted you needed it to make almond butter. Then it was the Jason Vales juicing – £200 quid on a juicer and almost £3k on his retreat that, thank God, the credit card company rejected"

I sigh and start Googling 'vegan celebrities' – but the rant is taking hold.

"Then remember the 5:2 when I had to pick you up from work at half four because you had fainted from hunger. And the Atkins when we became on first name terms with the butcher and he got his first holiday in years with the profits from our purchases"

This is all true, to be honest – but I know veganism is the way to go. I try to distract from the rant "Look – Ellie Goulding... Miley Cyrus... Ellen De Generes – they look amazing and are all vegan" I try to explain but to no avail. My partner is on verbal vomit mode and can't be stopped.

"Then that Powderdrink shite – £500 quid on packs of powder and where did that get you?". I am getting annoyed now "Yes – but I lost 15lbs," I say indignantly. And I did – ok I put 20lbs back on but I lost 15!

"Then the hypnosis sessions and having to listen to Paul McKenna telling us he could make us thin every bloody night"

It's time to interrupt and make a point. My partner though not as podgy as me has put on a few pounds lately. "Look at Kate and Jim down the road," I say triumphantly. "They are vegans and slim and healthy – we can be like that"

"Oh for fuck's sake" is the response. "Kate and Jim are thin because they run marathons every few weeks and have personal trainers. When you are out getting pissed with your pals and eating kebabs on the way home, Kate is in the gym working out. On Sunday mornings when we are hungover watching Corrie in bed with bacon sandwiches, Kate and Jim are doing wild swimming. That is why they are thin. Not because they are vegan"

I am getting strong vibes that I am losing this argument because of my partners over-reliance on factual information to back up their case. I try to think of a way to get the upper hand but my brain fog and the remains of a hangover is stopping me thinking as quickly as normal so I stay quiet trying to think of a smart final comment. Also, I can't get a bloody word in edgewise.

"Yes, and there is another thing – running – you bought that subscription to Running World and bought two pairs of very expensive trainers and a ton of running outfits. You then signed up to run 10k for that Donkeys in Greece charity thing – which can I remind you is only 3 weeks away – and so far you have only been out twice and still can't run more than 2k.

"And we still have cupboards full of that slim-your-tum shite from the last fad" Finally my partner stops for a breath. "I have successfully found a number of weight loss methods that do not work for me" I replied stiffly.

My partner is in a bit of shock as I am not arguing back – not realising I am trying not to laugh. Not used to having the upper hand they carry on full of hope that this 'fad' can be hit on the head. "And all your shoes – and those Michael Kors bags and purses... leather – so are you going to get rid of them? You will have to if you are going to be a VEGAN". I don't like the emphasis on vegan... as if it is a dirty word.

"You are right," I say – "I cannot be a hypocrite – the leather would have to go". My partner perks up sensing a victory. "The good news though" I continue" is that there are vegan equivalents – Mink... Matt & Natt... all suppliers of vegan shoes and handbags. And it is nearly my birthday... so it is a great opportunity to replace everything"

"What?" My partner is now sensing victory starting to slip away and not quite sure how it happened.

I feel a bit bad and say 'hold on – I'm off to get blindfolds – I have an idea'. I run and get the 2 eye masks we have in our kitchen shit drawer from a long haul flight a couple of years ago. I come back and cover mine and my partner's eyes with them. My partner is wide-eyed – could victory still be in sight – winning an argument and still in with a chance of getting it... that never usually happens,

But I beg to feckin differ. It isn't happening as something is much more important. I feel my way into my bag and pull out 5 different bars of vegan chocolate as I must have an alternate to Galaxy. Time for a blind tasting session. We are delighted to find that the 45p bar from Tesco is better than the £3.50 bar from Holland and Barratt. But we have to eat quite a lot to confirm those findings and it gets a little messy.

The dog walker returns with Sweet Dog to find us in the midst of piles of melting chocolate and blindfolds and gets very flustered (note to self must remember she has set of keys) and quickly excuses herself. Sweet dog goes nuts and tried desperately to get to the remaining chocolate. Partner goes off to walk her again while I tidy up the chocolate mess and put all our vegan stuff into the cupboards throwing out quite a bit of slimming world crap as I go to makes space.

Half an hour later they are both back... with Quorn bacon rashers!! On offer at Tesco apparently. And some squirty vegan ice cream. And a gleam in the eyes (of my partner – not the dog). Just as well I didn't throw the blindfolds in the washing machine!

I think this vegan thing will work out just fine.

CHAPTER 29

A rant about Snowflakes

In this chapter, I bring to you – my meno-rant on bloomin' Snowflakes!

OK so I know I should be grateful to Snowflakes – one day they will be paying for my pension/benefits/prison stay (depending on what old age option I go for and perhaps even wiping my arse when I get to that age.

But they are annoyingly young and fresh. I was at a 'training event' at work – won't bore you with the details but we had to all start by giving an interesting fact about ourselves that might surprise people. Well, I was most excited – I did a similar exercise about ten years ago and everyone was most impressed.

Finally it's my turn. 'I was on Top of the Pops dancing behind Craig McLachlan' I announce proudly. Blank looks all round. Too late, I remember the average age is around 28. I continually forget I am twice the age of half the people I work with. 'Who's Craig McLaughlin?' says the graduate snowflake. 'What's top of the pops?' says the Apprentice snowflake. 'FFS – It's Craig MCLACHLAN I', say then I sing a bit of the song 'Hey Mona... OOOO Mona' just in case it triggers a memory – but there is zero recognition. A sudden urge to get up and do the dance comes over me but I manage to resist and we move on to 24-year-old Snowflake Cliff who tells us about his climb up Kilimanjaro to raise £5000 for orphaned orangutans or something similar. When did young people get so bloody compassionate? Do none of them get wrecked on cheap booze while hanging out on street corners the way my generation did? The youth of today just don't know how to have fun.

Anyway – I resolve to find a more recent interesting fact in case I am in this position again.

At break time the Apprentice Snowflake approaches. She has checked YouTube and cannot find me dancing on Top Of The Pops. I explain that it was some time ago and YouTube wasn't around then. 'No YouTube' she says in wonder then glares at me again 'well do you have a picture?' 'No' I sigh and I can tell she is sure I am lying now – no selfie? So I have to give a short history lesson on how you used to have to take a proper camera out with you not just fish your phone out because shock horror – there were not mobiles!. And due to the likely vast intake of cheap booze you often didn't take it coz you would have broken it or lost it. And in actual fact, we often went out and... did not take one single photo all night!! I am getting into my stride when her apple watch makes a noise which tells her she must go and run up and down the stairs. I watch his retreating back and remember when we just did exercise without needing a bleep to tell us when to do it.

Anyway the day dragged on. At lunchtime the snowflakes blethered on about not being able to afford to move out of home. I tell them I did as I wanted freedom and a little cupboard with a mattress in a shared house was the only option so I took it. They look horrified. Finally, it was time to go home. I was most depressed as I wait at the bus stop – as I couldn't think of a single interesting anecdote about myself in the last decade. Not one!! I rack my brains. What happened? I've tons from before but I need to be more relevant for the next one. My mood is falling – a Snowflake 'yoof' joins the queue eating his pie from Greggs. Well, he eats half of it and throws the other half in the street. I don't know whether it is the menopause rage or if I am justified (it is often hard to tell?) but I am raging. 'Mate – you just dropped your pie on the road' I say. 'So?' he says in an insolent way. 'So it means you are a DIRTY FECKIN BASTARD' I say, 'Pick it up and put it in the FECKIN BIN which is conveniently situated just a 12-step walk from where you are standing'. He looks at me slack-mouthed. Snowflakes are not used to such a response. And I get a slight panic... Oh no... What have I done? In today's world does this mean I could be accused of being Snowflakist? No one else at the bus stop is menopausal and it is Edinburgh so they are all just pretending they haven't heard anything. I suspect if I am stabbed they will just step over me trying to avoid the blood and get on the bus. I see a taxi and quickly flag it down. Yes, I should be saving money but this is really a health and safety thing.

Back home and I search Spotify – there it is. I try my dance steps out – I can remember them!!! I dance around the living room ecstatic. I mean the steps were fairly easy – I just happened to be in the crowd and pulled up to do a simple dance with a few others – but I've still got it going on!!

I have a couple of drinks and open my laptop and check out skydiving; canyoning; Everest climbing and a number of other exciting but slightly scary activities. I have yet to choose – but I WILL have an exciting fact to share next time. Those snowflakes will see me for the exciting person I am.

But for now it is 9pm and time for bed!

CHAPTER 30

Nights out

In this chapter, I bring to you – my meno-musings on night out as a menopausal woman.

I had a night out a while back – one where I decided I would get all dressed up for a change. I haven't really been bothering my arse making much effort to look good lately. I made a half-hearted attempt last year and ironed my trousers and straightened my hair rather than putting on up in a scrunchie. But at the same time was googling to see if there were any restaurants that had a pyjama dress code. But I wandered past a window in town the other day and there was this fat scruffy messy woman who had the same colour hair as me. Discovering this was because it was actually me was a shock.

This is a 'proper' night out and might go on very late. I haven't had a proper night out in ages because menopausal wakefulness at 5am does not lend itself to any social event that prevents me being in bed by 10pm. Indeed cancelled plans are rapidly becoming my favourite kind of plans as a result of a few weeks of overestimating my capacity as a menopausal woman to party. Also, I can't hear a thing in all these trendy bars and I don't like standing all night. And taking my jacket off when I have a hot flush then holding it not really knowing what to do with it before putting it back on isn't fun. My favourite thing to do now is lunch – home by 7pm – have the hangover while I sleep. But I am on a bit of a high at the moment so think I am going to go for it.

It isn't possible to lose 3 stones in a day (much as I have tried) so I decided to make the most of everything else. Operation Gorgeous commenced. I am considering Botox but slightly scared so opted to have a fringe cut in which should have the same effect of hiding the wrinkles.

Ninety-eight quid later (note to self – go to wee hairdresser at end of road and pay £30 rather than pop into posh salon in George Street – fecks sake, they even charge for a cup of tea!) I leave and have to admit I am looking pretty fantastic. My wavy hair has been straightened to within an inch of its life and is swinging like a thick glossy curtain. But then it starts. NO NO NO. Not a hot flush. I stand as still as I possibly can. Please flush don't come. But it does. Hot flushes make me sweat through my head. Benefit is no underarm sweat patches or back sweat patches. Disadvantage is it makes my hair wave and tangle into a curly damp mess. Not in a tousled sexy way but in a matted laid in bed for three days kind of way. FOR FUCKS SAKE! I say out loud startling a lovely old woman who swerves her shopping trolley out the way to avoid me. Finally it passes and I rage on. Not paying ever again for a blow dry and may seriously consider a Sinead O'Connor look going forward.

Then it is time for my eyebrows which are quite fair and due to thyroid issues (often a joyous partner to the menopause) they are rather sparse at the ends. I go to the salon and make it EXPLICITLY clear the dye is to be on for no more than 15 seconds. I DO NOT want a repeat of last time where they looked fab in the dimly lit salon room then I nearly crashed the feckin car when I looked in the rear view mirror and two massive black caterpillars had appeared on my forehead. I am NOT part of the caterpillar brow generation – I do not want eyebrows that go from my tear duct to my lug! I had to take two days off work as could not go out in public – and rub them like crazy with wet wipes and eye make-up remover to make them look vaguely ok. The 12-year-old beautician looks blank – 'you need it on longer than that' she says. I know she isn't taking kindly to my commands but you can't be everyone's cup of tea. Otherwise you would be a mug. I saw that on a fridge magnet and it resonates. I mean I do try to be inspired by more highbrow quotes but this I think is a good one. And I don't' want to be a mug. So I reply very firmly NO I DON'T – getting old has its benefits in assertiveness. I need it on for 15 SECONDS. I will count out loud so we don't forget. And they do look rather dapper when done – exactly how they should be.

All is going well. I have a lost half a stone on my VLCD which means with a push and a shove I can get into a size 18 (never saw the day I would be glad to get my arse into a size 18 – remember being devastated when I moved into a size 12... FFS... was I mad??). I am a little excited about this because the next size down is a 16 which is the average for the UK – and I am taller than average at 5'7". This means that when I drop the next size I will officially be slimmer than average. This is good. So I get some lovely red stretchy capris trousers and a fab white shirt and some wedges. "How do I look?" I ask my partner. 'OK' is the response. Which is exactly what a girl wants to hear when she has spent the whole day getting ready.

I try to find my wedges. Fecks sake – where are they. Hunt hunt hunt. We have bought an Alexa and she can answer so many questions but I am now thinking a menopausal Alexa would be useful. And by that I mean one that aids menopausal women.

E.g. 'Alexa – where are my shoes?' 'They are in the fridge of course darling'. As opposed to a menopausal Alexa who would probably just say 'Find your own fucking shoes you half-wit'

I am driving so that I don't get drunk as trying to stick to the diet. Off I go with my shades on and looking fab, window down and singing along to Paloma Faith's version 'Play your own kind of music' on repeat and deciding that is now 'my song'. Then I hit the Kingston Bridge. The feckin cunty bastard bridge. Tailbacks forever. I sit and wait. And wait. Then disaster – my VLCD means drinking a LOT of water. And there can be no input with output. I am desperate. Really desperate. I search the car – anything at all I can pee into. Feck – tidied the car as read that decluttering helps with brain fog and now there is nothing to pee into. Am gonna find the name of that bloomin' author and give them a piece of my mind!. Oh no. I don't think I can wait. I quickly Google peeing in a traffic jam and I am gonna have to follow the advice. I open the back door and my door to create a private booth type area. Then carefully perch on the end of my seat and push my arse out slightly. And blessed relief. I pee and pee and pee and pee. It works. None on shoes none on clothes. Maybe someone did see me – the motorcyclist that whizzed up the hard shoulder perhaps – but literally don't care. I can breathe again. I spend the remainder of the time in the jam learning the lyrics to my new song – I think it takes about 19 plays which isn't bad when you are contending with menopausal brain fog.

Finally get to Shazza's and the wine if flowing. 'Just a diet coke' I say to Tina, who is in charge of drinks, feeling smug about my will power.

An hour later I am pissed on Rum and half a bottle of Chablis. Shazza/s husband says he will drive us as he is now desperate to get shot of us. Apparently there is some football tournament thing on he is keen to watch on telly.

We have quite a fab time and as we are twirling on the dance floor I catch sight of myself in the mirror. Looking not to dissimilar to the wanton mess that reflected back to me in the shop window yesterday. The young and the beautiful are reflected beside me snapping themselves on instasnapchat. I manage to photobomb a few of them. They will possibly delete the resulting snaps as I think it hangs them up to see someone like me.

But I don't care because I am following Mann and Weil's advice – making my own kind of music.

And singing my own special song.

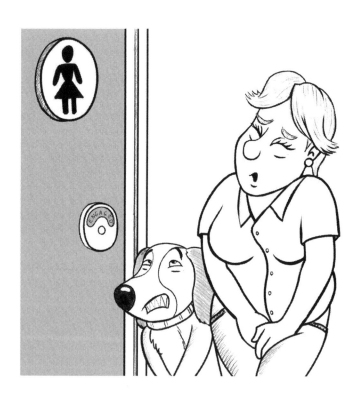

116

CHAPTER 31

Let's talk about sex

In this chapter, I bring to you – my meno-musings on sex (or more accurately – the lack of it...).

Well if menopause is taboo – and Sex is taboo. Then sex in the Menopause is the very lastest taboo in the whole universe!

I was going through puberty just as the AIDS epidemic hit and the scaremongering got me so anxious I was scared to even kiss anyone in case I caught it (how ridiculous). I was also very innocent. While others snogged their teddies for practice I rubbed my neck on mine as the kids at school called it 'necking' and I was a very literal kid. I have always had a tendency to be literal – I had a similar issue as I got older with the term 'blow job' but that's probably not something we need to go into.

If I am being really honest – I have considered just shutting up shop 'down there'. Not just closing for a refurb – I mean just closing it down for good. I'd just prefer to go to bed and sleep or watch documentaries on serial killers.

What the actual fuck happens to the 'down below' bits during the menopause?

To our 'foofoo's. Our 'snatches'. How many words are there out there for our vagina? A game I played over rum cocktails with some friends revealed at least fifty – fanny; beef curtains (!!); everyone's favourite 'c***''; beaver; punani; lady garden; lady bits; crotch; muff; snapper; ladyflower; twat; front bottoms... the list goes on. We mused over this – I mean we don't have 20 names for our arm or our foot do we? Anyway I digress

The libido just fucks off about this time. Like totally fucks off without even a goodbye text. I feel like getting a wee headstone and putting it in the bedroom 'in loving memory of my Libido – taken unexpectedly and before it's time'. I wish my browsing history in my phone had porn or maybe on-line sex shops but it is just puppy websites and orders from the local pizza place.

When I really really didn't want it at all ever ever and was seriously considering a career change to be a Nun, I decided I'd ask my oldest pal, Jessie Stopes, about it all. She is menopausal and gave me great advice on coping with it as she is a year or so ahead of me. I really wanted to have a good heart to heart. I don't see her often enough due to life getting in the way but we had a lunch planned. I was a bit late as I forget where we are meeting and need to scan through WhatsApp, then my texts, then my emails and finally find the location on Facebook (thankfully she is Facebook obsessed and checks in everywhere she goes – it is a big help). She is the same age as me – in fact, 2 months older! I am going to ask her and am looking forward to a long chat about improving our sex lives. We get wine and settle down and I ask how her sex life is since hitting the menopause. She almost drops her wine. 'We are in a restaurant' she whispers looking around in horror. 'But I just want to... I mean are you still doing it? I say... desperate to talk about it. 'No... no there are some things that are private' she says and then, 'Let's decide what we are having to eat'. I am dismissed. This is the woman who 30 years ago told me in great detail in McDonald's about her genital warts diagnosis and treatment while referring to the guy who gave her it as that 'fucking riddled cunty bastard' in a voice loud enough to be heard a mile away. And then she finished with her next partner and told me again in MacDonald's in a loud voice how we was odd as he kept pulling her pubic hair (in the days when we all had pubic hair... after having seen Naked Attraction it would appear that is as out of fashion as orange swirly carpets). We later found out that he has misheard her when she said she liked gentle hair pulling. But anyway – so now.... she can't bring herself to talk about sex during the menopause!! I am about to remind her of that story but I stop myself. I am finding myself in trouble a lot for not filtering what's in my head before it comes out my mouth. I think now is one of those moments where silence might be the best option.

My partner was a little down about all of this. It took a while for them to work things out as I used great avoidance techniques involving long walks, heavy meals and lots of wine which has a great sedative effect. But they started to get a bit wise to this. So I then suggested I sandpaper their bits so they can experience sex from a menopausal woman's perspective. They declined. So I declined too. Not having sex is becoming one of my great talents.

Feckin ironic given at long last it's a time that menopausal women can shag away with no chance (or little chance...) of pregnancy.

My fanny problems took me (again) to the Doctor when she said something about a Trophy. Yes, I think – Yes I do deserve a trophy. Or at least a bloody medal for putting up with this shit. But no – it was atrophy she said – which is very different. Basically our bits are dying off. Thickening and closing up.

I feel like a feckin science project. What next? Women should get compulsory trips to the Doctor were they tell you that your pubes will go grey; your fanny will dry up; you will want to stab lots of people; you will never want to shag again and your chin will soon resemble Desperate Dans. Then at least you will be prepared.

Bloody Tina is the opposite though – keeps telling me how horny she is. So maybe there is hope. But until then there is catch up telly and chocolate.

CHAPTER 32

Menopausal Love Island

In this chapter, I bring to you – my meno-musings on the telly programme 'Love Island'.

I was watching the last series and it got me thinking – what would it be like if they moved all the girls out and replaced them with menopausal women! I think it might go a bit like this:

Voice Over Man:

Welcome to Love Island. Sponsored by Incontinence Pads Inc.

Tensions are brewing in Paradise tonight as the 10 menopausal women brought in yesterday to replace the previous female contestants make their presence known.

We have to share the sad news that Jack has made the decision to leave the show. His experience of 3 years living with a menopausal mother is taken as an acceptable mitigating circumstance.

Big Mags is on the warpath.

Cut to the Island with most of the contestants sitting round the pool.

Big Mags appears from the house:

"Where the FUCK are my tweezers and my magnifying mirror"?

Wes and Jack are quivering slightly – Wes more so as he knows he broke the mirror yesterday when trying to make a fire with it and the sun and some paper thinking it would make him look all Bear Grylls and he might get his own TV series after the series. "we don't know honestly Mags – we don't. Your eyebrows look fine to us though Mags"

Big Mags:

"Not for my fucking eyebrows you twats – for the pubes on my chin."

Wes to Jack:

"Pubes? Do women have pubes? I thought it was just us blokes"

Jack:

"News to me mate – never seen a pube on any girl I've ever dated – not on their chin or anywhere".

Jack and Wes ponder this strange concept.

Charlie wanders down to join them rubbing his eyes with tiredness. He was paired with Lou last night. He had tried it on with her having heard a lot about 'Cougars' and their sexual prowess. But she had told him to piss off and if that wasn't bad enough he did not sleep a wink due to her nocturnal flatulence and snoring.

He is not the only one to have not slept. Sam is curled up on a sun lounger dozing and refusing to ever sleep in the same bed as Rose again. He has been to the Diary Room and shared his concerns. Just before he entered the Island he had completed a thesis on spontaneous combustion and explains it to the producer "it occurs by self-heating due to an increase in temperature due to exothermic internal reactions" he says " then it is followed by a thermal runaway then finally autoignition". The producer tries to be patient but has just discovered that the 90 packets of Maltesers he had stored away had disappeared and only the wrappers remain – and his assistant has told him that Rose and Lou have eaten them all and are showing no remorse. 'Can you get to the point, Sam?' he says as kindly as he can as he racks his brain to think where he can get 90 packets of Maltesers in time for the live special 'Who can stick the most Maltesers up Their Bumhole' competition in just 2 hours' time.

Sam is very concerned 'It's Rose – I think she is in danger of Spontaneous Human Combustion' he hisses. "Her body was well over 100 degrees last night on several occasions"

"Oh Fuck Off," says the producer making a mental note to edit his less than sympathetic response out. Sam is petulant and says he refuses to sleep in the same bed as someone who may ignite and set him on fire.

Big Mags is complaining about everything. Wes asks timidly why she doesn't just leave if she is so unhappy.

Big Mags tells him it's because she forgot to get a fucking pension and the appearance fee will mean she can afford beans to go with her toast. Wes isn't too sure what a pension is but feels it would be a mistake to ask.

Cut to Break.

Adverts for tweezers, magnifying mirrors, plus size clothes and vaginal moisturiser are shown

Voice Over Man:

Back to our Contestants. Jane is here to steal one of the menopausal woman's men.

Cut to the garden where the menopausal women look like they couldn't actually give a flying fuck.

Jane appears – she has been on HRT for 4 weeks and her libido has returned with vengeance.

Idris is keen to impress and starts to gyrate – 'Whassupppp' he says 'you so pretty – your gorjus' he says. He is determined to get some action and this normally works. Jane isn't interested. She has heard there is a Doctor and feels that at her time of a life a Doctor is of more use. So she chooses Alex and they pair off. Liz breathes a sigh of relief she can feck off with her appearance fee and get back to reality. She was starting to get really worried that her hormones would make her do something that might end up on the news.

Alex and Jane disappear and arrive back two hours later. Jane is dishevelled but has a smile as wide as the River Clyde and Alex looks shocked having learned more about a woman's body than he did in 7 years in medical school!

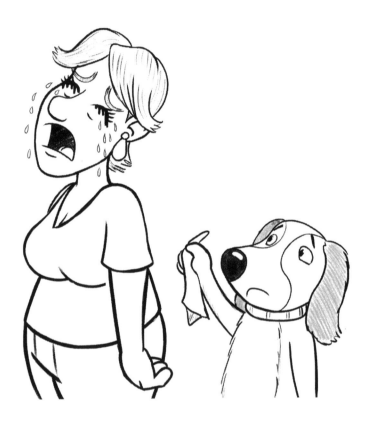

CHAPTER 33

It is absolutely OK
not to be OK

In this chapter, I bring to you – my meno-musings it being absolutely OK not to be OK!

I had this muse in Mental Health Week

It got me googling to find out the suicide rates in the UK – and one fact on the Office for National statistics page was a real shocker. The most common age for female suicide is 51-55 years. And what is the most common age for menopause? Yep 51-55 years! Is this just a coincidence? I Googled more trying to find any studies on the potential link – but nothing. Absolutely nothing. And I find that shocking.

Maybe there is no proven link, but let's face it – when you are entertaining anxiety, insomnia, low mood and irritability amongst others – is it any wonder that depression wants to pop along and join the party? Add to that the pressures women of our age can often be under – grown-up children leaving home (or not leaving home!!); not having children and realising you never will; caring for ailing parents; financial pressures; pension worries; realising that you are no longer young and suddenly being aware of just how much society values youth etc., etc. And you have the perfect storm.

There is no doubt that falling estrogen levels can affect your mood. The physical symptoms can also start to affect your mental health. Those hot flushes can lead to panic attacks and not wanting to go out in case they hit. The lack of sleep can make you feel down and make it hard to see things clearly. The irritability can make you start to alienate the very people you need around you – at one point I was telling so many people to fuck off that I worried I may have Tourettes!

Every woman is different – with different circumstances and different responses to the menopause. What will help one woman won't necessarily help another. What definitely doesn't help are stupid comments from half-wits that I sometimes read online such as:

- oh get on with it and stop making such a drama
- every woman goes through it – you're are no different
- it's just natural
- FFS – can you just stop going on about it – you're not the only one
- some people are so much worse off than you – just get on with it.

Bollocks – all bollocks – at this time of life it is absolutely OK to not be OK about everything that is going on in and around you.

Carol Vorderman has been honest and spoken out about experiencing suicidal thoughts and depression during the menopause. Gillian Anderson said she felt her life was falling apart around her and was completely overwhelmed. Lorraine Kelly has said she just didn't feel like herself and could not see joy in anything. And good on them for being so open – I think the more people that speak out – the easier it is for others to talk about it and start seeking help.

My niece asked me what the menopause was and I answered honestly – she thought about it for a while and then said – 'so it's all the rubbish bits about being a teenager but you are also old' So that fair cheered me up!! But it does kind of sum it up. On the flipside it can also be a time to fully evaluate your life and what you want to make the rest of it the best of it. Oprah Winfrey described it as your moment to reinvent yourself after focusing on the needs of others for so long – to get clear on what matters to you then to pursue it with all your energy time and talent. And once my savings account balance goes past £37.60 I will also recruit a personal trainer, therapist, life coach and go on lots of holidays and reinvent myself as Oprah.

There is no 'one size fits all' – every menopausal woman needs options tailored to themselves. Some women (very few) sail through without an issue, others experience minor symptoms and for others it is extreme. Apparently only 50% of women who suffer actually go and seek treatment – I'm not sure why that is. Maybe because not so long ago the hormone changes were seen as a sign of madness. Are women scared of putting it out there? Worrying if people will judge? Scared people will think less of them? Attitudes to mental health are changing (thank God) and there are a wide range of options the GP can discuss or refer you elsewhere when needed. There are tons of online forums where women are talking about their symptoms and supporting each other. The more we talk about it the less of a taboo it will become, so let's talk about it.

You are not alone.

CHAPTER 34

Menopausal exhaustion

In this chapter, I bring to you – my meno-musings on the wrecking ball that is menopausal exhaustion

I mused on this one of the many evenings I was tucked up in bed at 7.30pm. But don't judge me – I had 'The Menopausal Exhaustion' (the kind that hits with the force of a ten-ton truck!). I had a proper grown-up social life for nearly 2 weeks! Yep, my normal evenings of home; bra off; telly on have been abandoned due to an unusual boost of energy which may or may not be HRT related (2 months in and so far so good) and the Edinburgh Festival right on my doorstep. Hence going from social butterfly to cocoon.

And as we all know a hectic social life as a menopausal woman is a very different story than a hectic social life when you are not a menopausal woman. Indeed I may well have overestimated the menopausal woman's ability to party! I actually thought I could go out three nights in a row including one after work!! And not go to bed 'til 11pm!! It was all OK 'til I realised that meant putting clothes on and leaving the house. What was I thinking? Brain fog made me forget my complete inability to function unless in bed by 9.30pm

Firstly the fringe venues – tiny teeny tiny and SWELTERING!! I do not friggin need any help with keeping warm. The HRT has not cut the hot flushes. Laughed so hard at one event the sweat droplets landed on the man next to me – he was rather horrified but a true Edinburgh gent about it all. I also peed myself a little bit but think I got away with it.

And the seats! Designed for the arses of the likes of Victoria Beckham and Kylie Minogue. I do not have the arse for gold hot pants or for trying to perch on these tiny seats without spilling over onto the seats next to me. I remember dreading the fatso coming to sit beside me at events. Now I am that fatso. Feckin Karma... I can see them walking tomorrow going inside their heads 'please no – not beside her... please no... oh fuck it is!!'

And the way I always end up right along at the end of a row – with a bladder like mine this is not a good thing – Edinburgh people are generally polite though and pretend they don't mind getting up to let you out to the loo after 15 mins in especially when you stand on their feet and spill your drink on them!

And for some reason, although having achieved the superpower of invisibility to most since hitting menopause – I still seem to have no problem attracting the loonies at these events. I sometimes wonder if someone is having a sick joke and that my 'lady care' magnet is actually a 'looney magnet' and there is a secret camera watching. Coz if there is a looney (I do hope that isn't now a highly offensive un PC term – I am getting so confused with what can and can't be said these days) about when I am sat waiting for a show you can guarantee they will come and sit beside me. I've had the shouters, the drunks, the ones that find the concept of shutting up for an hour to actually listen to the feckin act an alien one. My supplements are helping reduce my desire to stab such people which is reassuring. I mean I still want to stab some people but probably the more deserving like the fuckwit on the bus that played some loud YouTube crap music video all the way from Stock-bridge to the Pleasance. I would have got away with mitigating circumstances on that one. Indeed an award for services to the community may well have been in order.

The tiredness also seems to make me clumsier. That night I was sporting a scraped arm where I fell down the stairs at one of the Fringe venues (while sober I may add!!); a bruise on my leg from walking into the side of a low table in a bar; a burn near my belly button where I pulled my jeans on from the tumble drier not realising the button was hotter than volcanic lava until I went to button them! A burn is also on my nipple from miscalculating the reach across my superduper new heated clothes horse to get a dry bra. I also have burnt fingers from peeling the lid off my microwave meal too early. Which I then stung on nettles when I reached into a bush to get some tasty early season blackberries. Then when I grabbed a dock leaf to soothe the sting, a wasp was under it and stung the tip of my finger. I mean you couldn't make this up. I am quite literally an accident waiting to happen. My partner is getting embarrassed due to the mildly accusing looks they get given when we are out. Which is ironic as the phrase 'wouldn't hurt a fly' applies quite literally to them – last night they took half an hour getting two flies out the bedroom... half an hour of gently cajoling and half a roll of Andrex tissue to set them free (to probably fly into some other half-inch crack to buzz all around their house).

As opposed to my approach which is to rush around the room with a rolled up magazine shouting 'DIE FUCKERS'

But life is for living... and while I am alive I am always gonna make a dive for the front seat!

Just as soon as I've watched Corrie in bed with a nice cup of tea and a Chocolate Digestive.

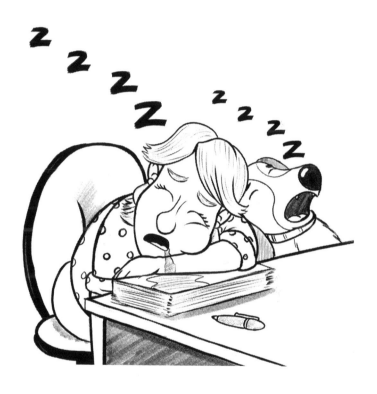

CHAPTER 35

Becoming a runner

In this chapter, I bring to you – my meno-musings on becoming a runner.

I spent a lot of time musing about being a runner. My partner and my pal Tina who runs a lot kept saying I should just put my trainers on and walk out the door and start running then I will be a runner rather than someone who just lies on the couch eating Maltesers while reading Runners World. This seems a rather simplistic approach but I do accept they may have a valid point.

So finally I did it – I chose the day for a number of factors. My Menopause book tells me that physical activity and exercise can relieve many of the common physical and mental/emotional symptoms that accompany 'the change' and I am very much in need of the 'runner's high' (tbh any high would do but running won't result in a stretch in Cornton Vale). I also need an out to vent the feelings that may otherwise lead to me punching random strangers for doing things like breathing too loudly or looking at me funny. Also, my friend who runs says if you run enough you can eat as much as you want because you burn it off which clinched the deal.

Also, while pissed on rum, I was persuaded by Tina to sign up for a 10k in June and now the cocktail induced cockiness has worn off I am slightly worried. Especially as we are doing it for charity so I can hardly just not bother to turn up without looking like a terrible person who doesn't care about saving Greek Donkeys

But on the positive side the 10K is 12 weeks away – so if I do the running thing and eat healthy foods then I will be 20lbs lighter and I picture myself floating gazelle-like over the finish line then holding my 10K medal high for photos that I can then post on Facebook and lots of people can say things like 'wow how fit are you?' and 'you look totes amazing!' instead of 'Feck that is a massive cocktail' and 'wow you look so well' which everyone knows means 'wow you have piled the beef on haven't you?'

Thankfully, as an organised person, my preparations are almost complete. So far I have:

- Downloaded Couch 2, 5K app on my phone

- Bought lovely white trainers in Run4It that cost a lot but come from a proper running shop so will be of very good quality and will make me run faster

- Gone back to Run4It and bought navy trainers as decided I did not want to get white trainers dirty by wearing them outside (white ones will not be wasted though as I am putting them aside for indoor use and will be using them when I get time to go to the gym I joined 6 months ago)

- Bought 2 lovely running outfits (not from a running shop as their idea of XL isn't mine – and also they think £18 is an OK price for socks)

- Drove past the meeting point for a running group but decided not to join them on account of being twice the size of the biggest man there and four times the size of the biggest woman

- Bought wireless earphones so I can run without getting tangled up

- Subscribed to Runner's World and been very inspired by the adverts of smart Activewear and the images of skinny runners

- Visualised crossing the London Marathon finishing line and being interviewed for Runner's World on how I had thought I was past it but now work as a Running Coach and attribute my new size 10 figure to my new lifestyle

- Bought two sports bras that are lovely and in time I may buy tops that will unbutton far enough that people can see the pattern of my sports bra peeking out. Actually if I get thin enough I might just wear my leggings and my sports bra when I go out running like some of the models in my magazine

- Been on Map My Walk and discovered some 5K routes around me that are off the road and quiet enough that few people will see me but not so isolated that I might get mugged

- Bought some special running sweets – 'running gels' to give me energy while I run.

So it was time! Time to run!

Sweet Dog was most excited and wagged her tail frantically in support when I put my trainers on so I couldn't bear to leave her behind. And also I had seen an article in Runner's World where a gorgeous slim woman was running with her dog beside her and I decided I wanted to portray a similar image. I also suspected I might be too knackered to walk her after my run.

So off we went. I drove to the park with the Loch that has a path round it that measures exactly 2.5K. Sweet Dog jumps out the boot and skips around happily. We set off at a nice gently slow jog. All is going well. My supportive bra is doing its job though to be honest I was at the back of the queue when they were giving out boobs so a vest would probably have been fine. My tummy swings from side to side which is a bit disconcerting but I soon get used to it swinging in rhythm with my steps. My arse is the most problematic as it seems to have got a life of its own and I seriously start to think of designing then pitching a 'bum bra' at the next Dragons Den.

Then Sweet Dog starts the Shit Twirl. FFS!! Thank God I brought poo bags. I am not to be put off so I scoop it up and run on trying not to boak when my hand comes up near my face (which they tend to do every few seconds when you are a Runner) and the stink of poo overcomes me. WTF does that dog eat? Two minutes later and another Shit Twirl. I now have a bag of dog shit in each hand. I try to think of them as weights.

Where the fuck is a dog poo bin for goodness sake? Or any bloody bin!

Then I notice Sweet Dog has fucked off into a bush and is struggling to drag something out from under it. Oh God – please not make it a baby squirrel or little bird. She emerges proud as punch with a Robinson's bottle of what I would like to think is diluted orange cordial but suspect due to its proximity to the road may be piss from some lazy bastard that could not be arsed stopping for a wee so just pissed in his bottle and fired it out the window of his vehicle.

Stupid Dog will not give the bottle up. So now I am running holding a bag of shit while the bloody dog runs beside me proudly holding the bottle of piss in her mouth. I am really concerned that the image I am projecting is not anything like any of the Runners World images I have pored over. I make a note to never ever ever bring Stupid Dog with me ever again. And I hope and pray I do not bump into my ex.

Finally I find a bin and lob the bag in and drag the bottle from Stupid Dog's mouth and fire it in – but not before a bit of what I really do hope is Robinson's Cordial leaks out from where her teeth have bit into the bottle and splashes on my new running trousers.

I keep going and suddenly my tummy cramps – oh God – I need to go. I need to go RIGHT NOW. What will I do? Oh God – I run behind a bush and do my own Shit Twirl. WTF was that – has my body gone into shock from moving? None of the Runners World articles mentioned this side effect (which I have since found is quite common and even has an official name – Runners Trots or Faecal Urgency if you want a more medical term). I stagger out feeling rather weak but secretly wondering if that will help with the weight loss. I also think I have now got something else in common with Paula Radcliff (apart from the running thing) and at least no one was there to broadcast it to the nation (I hope).

I am knackered now as I have been slowly running with just those few stops for nearly 8 minutes. So I decide to walk the rest of the way. Running World warns against overdoing it on your first few runs.

I will obviously need to build up a bit more stamina before the 10K.

And possibly shop for some Imodium!

CHAPTER 36

Menopausal weddings

In this chapter, I bring to you – my musings about the menopausal wedding.

So I spent my 20s attending weddings. My 30s cuddling lots of lovely new babies. My 40s supporting friends through divorces. And as I enter my fifth decade it looks like attending 2nd weddings is the new black!

But it is a very different matter attending a wedding when you are a menopausal woman then when you are a young hot 20 something. Take my experiences of attending my friend's marriage at the weekend.

Outfit Choice!! I used to look for the clingiest sexiest outfit possible. But not now. I had six months' notice of this wedding and had planned to lose 20 pounds for it – a jump on the scales; last week revealed just 25 pounds to go!! FFS! I put this down to pre-Minstrel tension (yes I didn't misspell that – self-medication on round circles of chocolate alleviates the perfect storm that is PMT and Peri-Menopause). I am also a bit skint from menopausal poverty (lady care magnets; supplements; holidays to cheer myself up and incontinence pads don't come cheap) so really wanted to avoid spending money. My partner helpfully said there must be something in the wardrobe given it is so full that everything falls on your head when you open it. So I decided to have a good look.

Three hours later and I have said Fuck; Cunt; Bastard more times than I've had hot dinners. I am a bit drunk as my partner knows that when this language ensues then the only solution is Jack Daniels and Coke and has been passing glasses through as I try and ram my body into clothes that have mysteriously shrunk. I have rammed everything that doesn't fit into black bags for the attic – to be brought down when I have lost four stone. I am left with three smock tops, three pairs of leggings, jeans that used to be very baggy but now look like skinnies and a couple of maxi dresses. All my lovely shoes are still there though – I love shoes – they don't abandon you just cos you are a bit chunkier.

So the conclusion is I have to shop. Off I go a bit pissed and clutching my credit card. A few hours later and I have something that will do. As long as no one sees my side view. Not bad from front but arse and tummy need their own postcodes and so side view not flattering!! I am most depressed (seriously forget personal shoppers – put menopause counsellors in these changing rooms to provide support when the size 18s won't feckin do up) but then I discover the Hats section. And the shoes section. Hats and shoes are nice. They are my friends. I get an amazing hat and some amazing tartan shoes and I am happy. Very skint now but the bride and groom said no presents and so, all in all, I think it balances out.

Off to the wedding and we try to remind ourselves of names of all the new partners that will be there. Menopausal brain fog means I find it hard enough to remember friends of 40 years standing let along new partners of a few years. We get to the hotel. My Hat!! My feckin Hat!! My glorious lovely Hat. It isn't there. FFS FFS FFS. I have forgotten it – this forgetfulness is doing my head in. I start to cry. My partner doesn't understand and refuses to drive 3 hours home to get it. So I cry some more 'til we decide if I get a nice up do at the hairdresser next to the hotel it will be a good compromise. Then even worse – I only have one bloody shoe. How's is this even possible. Fuck it – I will wear my blue sketchers – I think I can carry it off.

The wedding goes with a swing. There is one close call where I meet a frenemy, Fiona bloody Barbour, who cheerily tells me she is wearing the same outfit that she did on the bride's first wedding. She laughs joyously as she says she thinks she might even be lighter than she was then. 'how bloody wonderful for you' I say as sarcastically as I can before being dragged away to the rather stunning buffet. I am relieved to see there are a number of other fatties – there was an array of fat bellies in the weddings in our 20s but normally they were baby bumps – they now are the result of the menopausal midriff. That there are so many intol-erants now (lactose/gluten/animal) means that there is loads for the 'tolerate anythings' like me so I get stuck in – waste not want not and all that.

The first dance is a success – at the first wedding the bride was so pissed she ended up lying on the dance floor and ordering everyone just to dance round her. So this is a win.

Then it's a bit of boogying for all of us. OK so 'Hot Stuff' and 'This Girl is on Fire' have different connotations now – but I can still dance like no-one is watching. I start to wonder if the DJ is taking the piss when they follow that up with Katy Perrys 'you're hot then you're cold' and am about to address the issue when I am reminded I am a bit pre-menstrual and we had come to an agreement I would not 'address issues' when PMT and menopause collide. My frenemy comes over and starts banging on about her 'portfolio patchwork career' which despite being pissed I rapidly work out means 'can't hold down a job'. I lose interest and look at all the teenagers glued to their screens rather than round the back getting off with some unsuitable. I swear teenagers take more photos of themselves in 24 hours than I had taken of me in my entire childhood.

At 10pm we have a quick debate whether that is too early to go back to the hotel and sleep. I used to sneak out of the house to go to parties when I was a teenager. Now I sneak out of parties to go home. My social life is often planned to allow me to be in bed for 9.30pm as menopausal exhaustion kicks in then – these second weddings should really take account of this... maybe have brunch weddings or something. But then the slosh comes on – the song of all Scottish Weddings – so I dive in to lead the way – I am BRILLIANT at the slosh and the good thing is the more drunk I get the better I get at it!! We manage through to 11pm which is a huge win and stagger upstairs and are asleep by approximately 11.10pm.

Then it is time to head home – to find a forlorn tartan shoe on the driveway that is soaked through with rain. And a grumpy Sweet Dog who wanted to come too and is gutted to have been left behind. We snuggle up and look at the Facebook pictures of the wedding and frequently have to email people to take the fecking pictures of me looking a size 18 down. I mean I am a size 18 but really – there are ways and means of photographing round that – mainly taking shots from the boobs up.

CHAPTER 37

Fuck all fits

In this chapter, I bring to you – my musings about when Fuck all Fits.

Holidays time is when I often discover Fuck All fits – and it was no different this year. And I mean Fuck All. Even my swimsuit is tight – my lovely multi-coloured slinky swimsuit that fitted last year is too bloody tight. Gonna have to take my black speedo one I wear when I occasionally go swimming as REFUSE to buy another Fat Bastard swimsuit. It is just too stressful – the makers of swimsuits for fatties assume their customers must all have juggernaut sized tits. This is not the case. The one part of my body not expanding on an almost daily basis is my tits – so the boob bits on the swimsuits for fatties just flap down sadly like Sweet Dogs ears over my wee fried eggs (note to self – remember to lose three stones next year and then you will reclaim your toned athletic body. Yes I bloody know I said that last year. And the year before. But wine, chocolate and Catch up telly get in the way). Or possibly forget the swimming suit and agree to go the nudist beach my partner discovered was quite close by completely co-incidentally while claiming to be 'looking up possible historical day trips' on TripAdvisor

But maybe it's just as well that Fuck All fits as there is hardly any bloody room in the case for clothes.

Seriously – going on holiday as a menopausal woman is rather different from going on holiday as a non-menopausal woman – when it was simply a case of flinging a bikini, flip-flops and a couple of books into a case and heading off.

Rather more is needed when packing now. It is medication first. Feckin medication. I hate being a person who needs 'medication'. My thyroid is fecked (common side effect of menopause) so I need tablets for that (people say an underactive thyroid is a great diagnosis coz you will lose loads of weight when you start the tablets – well I beg to feckin differ – lying bastards!). Forgot them last time and spent the last three days of the holiday fast asleep as just could not function. Well, tbh, I was also totally fed up with my holiday companions – tolerance levels of a menopausal woman are low to say the least – and was fucked off with the way one of them sniffed and the way the other one laughed. So lying in bed snoozing and reading and ordering room service was a better alternative to stabbing them.

Then the supplements need to go in as they stop me telling strangers to fuck off. And some sellotape to keep the feckers attached to my arse as they have an annoying habit of falling off. Then the tube of gel for the rosacea which is all over my fecking face (also hormone related apparently). And my magnesium supplements and magnesium spray which helps me sleep (apart from between 3.16am and 4.45am but getting used to that now). Nurofen for the achy joints which are the latest gift from the menopause fairy. Earplugs essential to stop me starring in 'Banged up Abroad' for suffocating my partner at 3am for snoring. Tweezers to deal with the chin hair coz even though I have had full face 'threading'' done for the first time yesterday (successful upsell from the beautician who used a lit mirror to prove that I was actually more Gorilla than Human). Hurts like feck btw – apologies to the person after me as my gasps of utter agony and less than strong pelvic floor meant occasional lapses in bladder control) I know for a fact the bright sunlight will encourage the little fuckers to grow loud and proud and show themselves off to the world.

Fanny magnet as can't wear it coz last time it set off the buzzer thing at security and I had to have a very complicated conversation with the not exactly empathetic guard who was most confused why my fanny beeped every time she ran the wand thing over it. Sanitary protection because though I am not due – the joys of peri menopause and HRT mean that I could have the painters in at any random time. Specs packed as arms no longer stretch long enough to read small print or even medium print. iPad with Homeland episodes downloaded to watch between 3.16am and 4.45am each morning.

So just room for a couple of kaftans. I put all my shoes in my partner's case when they are not looking – easy as they are glued to the iPad trying to figure out the best route to the airport. (it will be the tram as the stop is four minutes' walk and will take us straight there but why stop their fun searching various bus routes and Uber prices and last minute car parking charges). I like shoes – they don't take it personally if you gain weight unlike my feckin multi-coloured swimsuit!!

Then have a panic as think passport may be out of date. Then have bigger panic when can't find the bloody thing. Menopausal Brain fog means I can't find my driving licence either. Finally find them in my sock drawer (not been wearing socks for ages as so warm so no wonder I had no recollection). Passport is fine – six months to go – hooray! I look at the lovely non menopausal me starting back from the back page. I remember laughing when my friend said I'd be nearly 50 when I got a new one. Coz obviously that was so so long away – so so so long away that it would never come. Aye right... it was like hitting black ice and spiralling out of control towards the next feckin decade. I have to sit down for a minute when realise I will be nearly 60 when the next one is due. And it only took five minutes to get from 40-50.

Then relax. I am realistic and recognise I won't lose three stones by tomorrow so may as well have a big bar of chocolate and a cup of tea and watch telly.

Except... feck... feck... sunglasses. My posh designer sunglasses – bought for a ridiculous amount of money when I was on a menopausal high... Where are they!!!

ARGHGHGHGHGHGHGHGHGHG!!

CHAPTER 38

Trying the VLCD

In this chapter, I bring to you – my musings on the Very Low Calorie Diet.

Because I have decided that a VLCD (Very Low Calorie Diet) is the way to go to shift this menopausal beef.

I used to think it was a really unhealthy way to lose weight but I watched a thing on the telly last week that seemed to suggest otherwise. And my pal kindly said that it would be OK for me to do it as I am obese as opposed to just overweight. I can't argue as everything about me is getting bigger. So that and studying the before and after pictures of celebrities who have done a VLCD concluded my research. (though tbh I would have been v happy looking like their 'before' pictures)

Everyone knows being a fatso isn't good at any time but especially so in the menopause years when the fat migrates to your belly and thus gives far greater health risks than if it were more evenly distributed around your frame. And you have a tendency to low moods anyway and this is made much worse by having to shop in the plus size lines.

I just can't be arsed with the one pound off... half a pound off stuff. And I am a woman of extremes. So decided to give this a go.

I found my 'Consultant' by searching on the website for someone that looked like me. Bingo. Found someone that was the same height as me and started when she was two stone heavier than me. She is now 3 stone lighter than me and looks exactly like I want to look. Even her frame is similar to me.

So I rock up to the office fully focussed and determined. I was going to get all the stuff then head to Tesco for a last binge fest before kicking off (sometimes I do wonder if all these pre-diet pigouts are actually responsible for my fatness)

The first surprise was that the woman bore a lot more resemblance to her 'before' picture than the 'after' one. I am pretty sure she is heavier than I am now. I am not sure how I feel about this. Isn't this the equivalent of turning up to AA and finding the leader is drunk? But I am too British to comment.

I get weighed and she proclaims me fat enough to go on the diet. I listen to all the mumbo jumbo then choose my products. Lots of powders and bars. Sixty quid later and I am ready to go.

But I haven't got a bag!! Totally forgot – and I am really wanting to save the bloomin' planet but once again I have forgotten. No worries my Consultant says – I have a nice big plastic one here. Yes she does – a huge brightly coloured plastic bag festooned with the name of the diet company.

'Um – don't you have any others' I ask rather shyly. 'Nope,' she says cheerily. FFS – so I have to march through town clutching my bag that proclaims to the world I am a fatso and on a major crash diet. Does she know the areas I have to walk through on my way home? Then I remember – Tesco – I can hardly go in there for my last big pig out and put my cakes and biscuits and curry into this bag – it would be mortifying.

So I find a quiet spot and pull everything out – turn the carrier bag inside out and refill it. Then I twirl it tight at the top – round and round. That's better – I can walk without embarrassment.

I buy a few wee treats as my final hurrah before 12 weeks of powder and shakes. I buy a nice big hessian bag and put my VLCD stuff in the bottom. Then I take them back and scoff them while I read the small print for my new diet. It would appear that nausea, hair loss and bad breath are possibilities. But for the degree of weight loss they promise – that seems to be a small price to pay.

I start my first day full of promise. I decide to have what the consultant described as a lovely cold chocolate milkshake. Except there is no chocolate. And there is no milk. And it isn't lovely. So I beg to feckin differ. It is powder with water. And the powder is all clumpy and lumpy. And it tastes disgusting. OK – VLCD Consultants – I challenge you to take a big glass of cold full-fat milk – add some hot chocolate powder (proper stuff – none of your options shite) and a huge scoop of chocolate ice cream and shove it in a blender. WHIZZZZ. Then when done put some scooshy cream on the top with a crumbled flake on top of that. Trust me – your shake ain't ever gonna win a taste challenge against that.

Oh well – off to work and I take my bar with me for lunch. It looks most forlorn in my bag but it will have to do. I am a little worried about the evening as I am off out with friends. My consultant said it would be fine to take a powder and tell the kitchen to make it up for me. I suspect that may have as much truth as the 'just like a chocolate shake' comment. Maybe Madonna can have chefs whisk up her special meals at the Chiltern Firehouse but I can't see Pizza

Express doing it tbh. I decide to consult the Facebook page I have been added to for advice. Before I do so I delete off the various slimming apps I was a member of before realising that VLCD was the way forward.

Hmm – the advice, in general, seems to be just don't go out and instead go home and have a bath and an early night. I can't not go out for 12 weeks! I read through more of the comments. 'Just order water and say you ate earlier' says Mary who has lost 19lbs and looks slimmer but sadder in her after picture. Well I am gonna look a complete fanny if I do that – 'oh yes I knew I was coming out for dinner so decided to eat before I came'.

I decide it is my first night so I won't have booze or pudding and choose a salad.

And I pretty much stick to that apart from just one glass of wine, a side order of chips and half of my friend's sticky toffee pudding with ice cream. But apart from that I did well. I go home after a couple of hours because generally speaking when people are pissed they talk shite. Which is fine when you are also pissed and talking shite but not so much when you are sober. I may have to get some new teetotal friends.

You have to drink loads and loads of water. I am finding that a challenge. Up 'til now I only found water tasty if I woke up with a raging hangover. Then it is the most beautiful gorgeous drink in the entire world. But – when I am sober – it is just meh!

But I am a trier – so I bought my big water bottle that says things like 'oh keep drinking' and 'well done half way there' to encourage you and feel well cool stoating about to meetings swinging it like all the other health-conscious people. I hadn't paid much attention before but some people's water bottles are MASSIVE and I am starting to pick up on water bottle envy. Who knew a water bottle could be a fashion statement. Also – drinking a lot of water has other problems. There is no input without output. I have to go to the toilet a LOT.

The week progresses with me working my way through the products. Here is my helpful guide to some of them:

Lovely Porridge – billed as a 'delicious option to have any time of the day'. If you want an idea of what it tastes like – mix some wallpaper paste with water and you will have the consistency about right.

Bangin Bolognese – billed as a 'classic Italian dish'. Well it is feck all 'like your mama used to make'. If you have ever had bolognese then threw it up, then eaten the vomit, then thrown it up again – I would imagine it tastes a bit like this.

Hot & Tasty Couscous – billed as a 'truly authentic dish'. Well it is authentically disgusting but the consolation is that it is so spicy that your mouth will burn so much you probably won't notice.

Chicken and Mushroom Soup – billed as 'warm and inviting' Hmm, about as inviting as a runny dog turd.

Macaroni Cheese – billed as a 'mouth-watering classic'. Just don't. GADZ! Trust me – just don't!!

Vanilla Rice Desert – billed as 'fluffy light with a delicious vanilla undertone'. See comments on lovely porridge above.

Bars – billed as a 'lovely naughty chocolatey treat'. Nope – a Galaxy bar is a lovely chocolatey treat. These are cardboardy yuckiness.

You get the picture.

It is weigh in tomorrow. And I am not sure I can carry on with it tbh – I stuck it coz had spent £60 on the stuff and had no money left for real food. Well when I say stuck it – I mean apart from the extra things in Pizza Express and a packet of prawn cocktail crisps and a few of my partner's chips. And a slice of birthday cake at work because it would have been rude not to. And a Jack Daniels. And a Glayva. Apart from that I have been spot on.

I have worked out that if I had a mars bar and a packet of crisps and a Freddo Frog every day that would be about the same in calories as this stuff.

Not nutritionally sound perhaps but much tastier.

CHAPTER 39

Shopping as a menopausal woman

In this chapter I bring to you, my musings on Shopping as a Menopausal Woman.

My musings started when I consulted my weight loss spreadsheet I set up 6 weeks ago when I decided to lose 44lbs so I could be classed as overweight rather than obese. After various calculations it turns out I now have 50lbs to go! I am good at sums but even if you aren't – you can tell this is not exactly a success story. My underactive thyroid diagnosis with the related medication was supposed to spur on my weight loss – but despite monitoring things closely by jumping on the scales six or seven times a day – nothing! Nada!!. Am fecking raging – and a little concerned as have Googled more on an underactive thyroid and it appears it is not simply a cause for celebration and weight loss as I had originally thought.

More googling tells me that it is the Menopausal Monster who has some responsibility for stealing my figure as well as my sanity (it is possible my addiction to wine and chocolate has also contributed – but let's face it, if losing weight was as simple as giving those things up then we'd all be bloody doing it!). Apparently lower estrogen levels make gaining weight much more likely – and also changes the distribution of weight as the fat all gathers round your belly in the menopausal years. Well, I could be the feckin perfect case study for that!!! I was blessed (and I could cry with how much I took it for granted) by being fairly slim 'til I hit my forties. I did get fat once for a few months when I was much younger after a particularly pleasurable 6 months in the States living off pizza and ice cream. I came home with a pot belly and was so upset about it (despite the fact I was still three stone lighter than I am now) but one benefit was that so many people would gave up their seat for me on trains and buses believing I was pregnant. On one memorable occasion I got upgraded to first class on a mobbed train as the guard said he could not leave someone in 'my condition' sitting on the floor. It was slightly marred by the fact I could not take advantage of the free alcohol being served as I feared disapproving looks when I was younger (don't give a shit now though – in fact I almost revel in them). But now I am way beyond childbearing age and my this combined with my invisibility as a middle-aged woman means I don't even get this benefit. I just look like a fat woman who ate all the pies and then all the chocolate bars.

I am further thwarted by snow that suddenly appeared and effectively turned me housebound. Can't get to the supermarket for fruit and veg so having to live off kebabs and chips from the place at the end of the road supplemented by some galaxies from the local newsagent. Two of the very few places still open and both owners probably planning a few weeks in a five-star hotel in the Maldives once the weather passes.

But I cannot give up. You see – they are knocking my school down. And they are doing an open day in 3 weeks' time for a last look round and loads of my old classmates that I haven't seen for over 30 years are going. My pal from school asked me to go but I said 'No' coz I feckin hated school. Plus I was pipe cleaner skinny at school and now I am a blancmange. And I don't want everyone saying – 'oh look at her can you believe what a fat arse she has now?' Or 'feck how did she get pregnant at her age – HAS to be bloody twins, maybe even triplets'. But then the Facebook posts and groups started and FOMO (Fear of Missing Out) struck. Also, my pal who is in touch with loads of people from school emailed me a list of all the ones she knew who were fatter than me, and it was quite a big list. I got her to cut and paste some of their photos from Facebook just to makes sure she wasn't lying – and it's true – a number do look rather chunky!. So now I am going. And I will just make sure I stand beside the Chunksters for photos coz that will make me look much slimmer than I am.

I have accepted that I won't be skinny in 3 weeks. Indeed empirical evidence suggests I may be even fatter than I am now. But a new outfit may just make me look cool for school. So I decided yesterday when we were sent home from work due to the snow (hooray) to stop and find a trendy outfit. One like I saw this cool girl on the bus wear. Jeans... Big Biker Boots... plain white top... and a nice smart leather jacket... gorgeous tousled hair. I watched her in awe 'til I noticed she could see a reflection of me staring at her in the window and was looking a little concerned for her safety.

My usual outfit since hitting my menopausal years has been leggings and a flowery smock – bought usually from the Super-market as I do the shopping. And I have to be honest – I have fallen into a bit of a rut in terms of making an effort. Not quite at the going to the Kebab shop in my pyjamas stage – but starting to feel like I have gone the extra mile if I go to work with my hair down. (Always with a scrunchie inside my bag though in case I get the sweats and have to tie it up after blasting it dry under the hand driers in the toilet). But I truly believe this is not me. There is a cool girl like on the bus that is just screaming to get out. (Actually, it is possible there may be three or four of them).

Suffice to say I did not enjoy my shopping trip. Hot flushes are not good when you are trying clothes on and mortified that you may have to hand the clothes back all covered in sweat... Stupid changing rooms where the curtains don't shut properly and all the young and the beautiful can see you're not so young and beautiful body as they walk past and the rooms are too bloody small – so your arse sticks out through the flimsy curtains as you bend to pull jeans on. Couple that with an irritable disposition and it all gets rather messy.

Shops need to cater more for the menopausal woman. Toilets in the shop for the continual need to pee isn't much to ask. Maybe some nice tunes from the 80s instead of the utter shite that passes for music these days. A quota of sales assistants must be over 40 or above a size 16. Feckin sizes need to go up way higher than a 16 too. Those bottle things that spray cool Evian water should be in each cubicle. And maybe a wine dispenser too. And some beds to take a short nap on when the exertions of taking clothes on and off combined with menopausal fatigue get too much. And maybe most importantly – a therapist within each changing area. There could be a button like in the posh shops that you press for another size, but this one is an urgent alert for that therapist to rush to the cubicle and support you as you sob at the loss of your tiny slim firm body that you never feckin appreciated at the time. It is true – you don't know what you have 'til it is bloody gone.

I did get my biker boots but they are the wide fitting ones from Marks and Spencer and strictly speaking not really biker ones – but they have a big buckle on them so I don't think anyone will be able to tell.

And I discovered pregnancy jeans!!!! They are great – perfect for the menopausal middle.

And a nice loose smock over the top covers that elasticated waist perfectly!

CHAPTER 40

Back to school

So in this chapter, I bring to you – my musings on going back to School.

My musings started as I planned to head back to school after 32 years absence!! My old school was being knocked down and to 'celebrate' they held a big open day with free cake and tea.

I wasn't going to go on account of being fat and also hating every minute when I was forced to go – so not seeing the point of going today when I actually had a choice.

But to be honest they had me at 'free cake'. And after seeing some Facebook pictures of other ex-pupils that were fatter than me. And I wanted to have good Facebook posts with me and my friends sitting at school desks. And I really wanted to draw on the chalkboards (I had originally written Blackboard but my pal's teacher daughter said that was now racist so it is a chalkboard. I am a little confused as it is black and it is a board... But I keep quiet because I got into trouble a little while ago at work for talking about brain-storming which is apparently offensive to epileptics and I was to use 'thought shower' in future. And I am trying to avoid turning into one of those people who are ignorant and offensive without meaning to be. Coz God knows my hormonal rages make me offensive enough as it is!),

I went to my mums first to make 'going to school' as realistic as possible. First shock of the day – thought I was looking pretty passible 'til I went to my Mum's loo. She has had a new magnifying mirror put into the bathroom. The bathroom that faces directly into the sunlight. A cursory look turned to a shocked stare as I realised I had turned into Desperate Dan. Ten minutes with the tweezers had me looking relatively OK again – but it was a near miss!!! I remember how we used to slag Mrs Beardy Bain from Maths – feckin Karma!! Another parallel – though 32 years ago I would have been in front of the mirror squeezing spot after spot then dabbing the latest Clearasil product on them before carefully arranging my hair to cover as much of my face as possible before heading to school.

Then my old school pals came over clutching some Buckfast to make things as realistic as possible. Which got me wondering if maybe the school will have organised any real-life events to make us really feel like we were back there. The Nimmo brothers waiting with eggs to pelt us with? Fights set up so we could all gather round shouting FIGHT FIGHT FIGHT? Semolina in the canteen?

We tried the Buckfast and much as we wanted to recreate the experience it tasted so disgusting we just couldn't. My mum reminded kindly that when we were 15 we had decades to enjoy good wine but now our lives are too short for crap wine. She then gave us 4 bottles of excellent Chablis then decided to leave us to it due to the ever-increasing volume of Simple Minds which we decided we MUST play before we went.

'COME IN, COME OUT OF THE RAIN', we yelled dancing around. I remember dancing at the school disco – I was just a wee blank dancing canvas so pretty much tried to copy the moves of the most popular girls there. But now I have my own style which has been described as 'unique and energetic'. But I am not offended as it is totally my style. Well – tbh – maybe modelled a bit on Beyoncé but what woman hasn't played Single Ladies over and over on YouTube 'til they had the moves down pat?

We then have a great idea – why don't we dress up as school girls and recreate Hit Me One More Time by Britney down one of the corridors. We think this is a great idea and quickly text our HWABG (Husbands Wives and Boyfriends and Girlfriends) to see if they could get us some uniforms for lardy chicks. But then we debate – perhaps this is not really politically correct. So we decide to just do the dance and text all the HWABG to tell them not to bother – Rosie's husband Chris is gutted as he was halfway to Primark to pick them up – but they will just have to live with it. We film ourselves doing the dance and send it to them as a kind of consolation. Though having watched the video and reflected – a large amount of Viagra would be required to turn anyone on after watching that!!

We are getting a bit tired with the dancing so it's time to slow it down with DON'T YOU FORGET ABOUT ME? Which made us sad but happy that we hadn't forgotten about each other. So we had to hug a lot apart from Fee who was having a hot flush and told us all to fuck off. Then we had to cry for a wee while too while we tried to remember all the pupils we had forgotten about despite promising at the school disco we would never ever forget them. Like EVER! Then we remembered the ones at school who didn't make it to this day. And we cry a bit more.

Slight panic then ensued as we realised the open day was going to finish in half an hour. So we all launched ourselves down to the school. Running late as always – but not quite as fit as we were and too pissed to drive so we were pretty knackered and sweaty when we got there.

And in we went with so many more parallels from our younger years. We were a mass of hormones there – and here we are again, slave to those strange things called hormones that control us like we are puppets on strings sometimes. We met Sad Sandy first who was always miserable at school. He attached himself to us and wandered around woefully talking about how he hated it here. We wandered from classroom to classroom sharing memories. We remembered the belt – and all felt it unbelievable that in our lifetimes it was perfectly legal for a 6-foot powerful man to take a tiny child and belt them pretty much on a whim. Sandy shook his head sadly – 'Mr Fletcher was the worst' he said 'I wish I could meet him now'.

"Would you punch him in the face?' I asked. Sandy looked at me 'No – it's just that I am really into S&M now'. I am never sure if Sad Sandy is making a joke or not as he never smiles so I make a noise that is a cross between understanding and laughing. Thankfully Katy decides we should now run through the corridors the wrong way as there are no prefects to yell at us to go the right way and to WALK! We actually only run a few steps because we are knackered and starting to feel the effects of the wine in our legs. Then we go the right way because we are really quite sensible and are getting in peoples way (and slightly afraid that someone might give us a detention).

I am impressed with my ability to remember almost all my teachers' names. Especially considering brain fog means I can't remember what I had for breakfast and nowadays I forget the name of just about everyone I meet within 5 mins of meeting them!

We go to the PE Changing rooms which resemble something from Train Spotting so we make a hasty departure but fondly recall Rough as Feck Rachel piercing Softie Sophie's ear with a bit of potato and a needle in there and her parents having to come and pick her up after she fainted. They took her to the Chemist in town to get the other one done – and tbh no one could tell which was which such was Rough as Feck Rachel's skill with her ear piercing tools.

And finally we get to the cake stall. Or at least what was the cake stall!!!! We were too late – all the cakes were gone!! Such was our devastation that two of the teachers who were running the tours gave us some celebration chocolates which helped a bit.

We were going to go on and get really pissed in the pubs we used to frequent with our fake ID when we were younger but tbh we were pretty exhausted after the excitement of the day and we all decided to go to our respective homes to watch Saturday Night Take Away with Ant and Dec after picking an Indian up on the way home. Just like our parents used to do... (though it might have been Morecambe and Wise then... hard to remember a time when there was no Ant and Dec...).

CHAPTER 41

Why this book is better than any other menopause books

In this chapter, I bring to you – my musings on the other Menopause Books out there – and why you made the right decision to buy this one.

You can't judge a book by its cover – so the saying goes.

There are lies damned lies and books about the menopause – so the menopausal women's saying goes.

I tried several High Street stores for a book on the menopause. I was raging and sweating when I got there. I had forgotten where it was despite having been there several times in the last few months. I reassure myself that at least I know now (thanks to Google) that this is a symptom of the menopause and not Alzheimer's (which incidentally I aced the test for at the doctors – defo not Alzheimer's!!). For the last year I thought I was going mad – I would get calls from friends asking where I was – I'd just totally forgotten to meet them. At work I'd be halfway through a meeting and realise I'd forgotten what happened at the start of the meeting. I'd get halfway through a book and forget what happened at the start. I regularly got lost travelling to familiar destinations. I was sweating just because that happens all the bloody time despite having done zilch exercise but walk 200 yards from car to the shop. I was raging because I had caught sight of my reflection looking a lot more like Jean then Helen Mirren.

Found the health and self-help section no problem as I had regularly visited it over the last year desperately looking for new meaning in my life. But never to find books on the menopause. But yet here I am. And there is nothing. NOTHING! That's right – NOTHING. I am now more raging. (I have been getting raging a lot over the last year). I can find out how angels can help my life. I can discover the power of crystals. I can even learn a bit about the Kama Sutra. Apparently I can make myself happy, feel the fear and do it anyway, cleanse my aura, learn the rules of love and get slim on a million different diets. But I cannot find out about the menopause. The sales assistant (male and about 20) is 'working' i.e. reading books on cars nearby. But I can't bring myself to ask. I scan the shelves again – every woman in the country will go through this – surely there is a demand for books on the topic.

And I need answers to a number of questions. So I decide to look online for a book to help me. And am surprised. But not pleasantly so...

It's the covers. If they are to be believed then the menopause is a time when your hair will become thick, shiny and glossy. You will have a wide smile showing even white teeth. Your body will be slim and lithe. According to one cover, when you enter the menopause your husband will start giving you piggybacks through meadows while you both laugh gleefully. One even referred to the menopausal years as the 'sexy years'. This made me laugh so much I weed myself a bit.

Well menopause authors.... ...I beg to feck in differ!!!

Menopausal women do not tend to have glossy hair, cheery smiles and have piggybacks from their partners before a rampant sex session. On account of their hair falling out, grumpiness, weight gain and diminishing libido.

Also the titles... titles like 'The Wisdom of Menopause'. Seriously! Trust me... you do not get wiser with the menopause. You get thick... thick as mince!!

And this for me is one of the worst things. I was the smart one of my friends when growing up. It was my 'thing'. My 'tag'. There was the 'wild one', the 'pretty one' and the 'quiet one' (though it turned out the quiet one wasn't as quiet as we discovered when we visited her in the wee Highland village she settled in. Suffice to say that the weekend we spent there proved that old adage 'the quiet ones are the worst' and that everything that happened in that village that weekend we agreed will stay in there unless the 'not so quiet one' decides to do her own blog – and trust me it would be worth a read if she ever does!).

Anyway back to the point (menopausal women waver from the point quite a lot – deal with it!!). I was the 'smart' one. I was. I've got a degree and a post-grad degree to prove it. I used to be able to absorb things quickly and could beat an elephant hands down in memory games. Not now. Now I forget everything. Everything. I can't remember if I cleaned my teeth... if I rinsed the conditioner out my hair... if I turned the straighteners off. The straighteners' one is a biggie. I now have to take a photo of the plug socket so that I can refer to it when inevitably I panic and think I have left it on after I have left the house.

I used to read books - loads of books - one after the other, devouring and getting lost in every single one. But in the last year I have read just two - I just don't seem to have the focus or concentration. As I type just now there is thick fog outside. Pea Soup weather as my Granny used to call it. Pea Soup brain is what I have.

Anyway - back to the books. I have ordered one of the books. Menopause for Dummies.

I am keen to find out:

- Should I have HRT? What are the benefits? What are the side effects? What happens when you come off it?

- If I had a hysterectomy - would that get it all over and done with? Or do you still have to go through it all?

- What are the natural alternatives to HRT?

- What is the longest time anyone has ever taken to go through the menopause?

- How can you tell how long it will take you?

- If you were to commit a crime, would being in menopause be considered a 'mitigating circumstance'.

And these books don't seem to hit the money at all. And they aren't even a little bit funny! So well done - you made the right decision to spend your hard earned cash on this one.

CHAPTER 42

Therapy

In this chapter, I bring to you – my meno-musings on going for therapy.

I am officially 'in therapy'. A decade or so ago 'coming out' in this way would have resulted in me being branded a Fruit Loop. But fortunately things have moved on. My aunt declares they have moved on too much and uses the example of the kids in school that now get therapy if the curly fries run out before they get to the front of the canteen queue. I am not sure of the accuracy of this but mental health does seem to be much higher profile now and for that I am grateful.

So what prompted this? Well, I went for my HRT check-up at the menopause clinic. A 30 min session that lasted 90 mins due to very very very high blood pressure. Which the doctor was concerned kept getting higher every 15 mins when they retook it. This may have been because I was anxiously checking with Dr Google between checks and realising a stroke or heart failure was just round the corner.

Anyway – upshot is I may have to go back to au naturel methods. And while I can just about cope with the physical symptoms, the biggest fear (from me/friends/partner/dogs amongst others) is the emotional turmoil. I searched through the alternatives to HRT, skipping past the daily Kale Smoothie/Spoon of Hemp oil etc and landed on CBT – Cognitive Based Therapy (be careful if you search that on twitter – apparently it is also a service some sadomaso-chistic men are looking for – the T stands for Torture – I'll let you work out the C&B... Who bloody knew!!).

I had a short term relationship about 30 years ago with a psychiatrist and it has always put me off a bit – especially the night out with their esteemed colleagues. All were totally utterly bonkers. It was bit like going out with a Al Anon group while they all got pissed out their heads.

But then in the Summer a friend had a spare ticket for Susie Orbach at the Edinburgh Book Festival and so I tagged along. She was the antithesis of the ex – cool, calm collected and giving an aura of 'I will fix you'. And she wore the most amazing sparkly shoes.

The psycho glitterati were asking highly complex questions so I did not feel able to ask about the glittery shoes. I did whisper to my friend if it was appropriate but got a hard long stare so I took this as a No. But I tweeted after and she replied telling me where to get them.

So, on this admittedly rather flimsy evidence of her credentials, I looked her up and although it said fee negotiable, I'm not sure I could persuade her to drop as low as £2.45 which is all I could afford as she is in London so I'd also have to pick up the commuting costs from Edinburgh. So I had a wee listen to her podcasts instead. She seemed to say 'hmmm' and 'ummmm' and 'uhu' a lot. So at least I know what to expect.

So decided to look a bit closer to home. Feck – it is a minefield. First the cost – £75 an hour seems standard! That's 3 bottles of Jack Daniels and a massive Galaxy – and I know for a fact they make me feel better. Therapy is more of an unknown.

I draw up a list of non-negotiable criteria to narrow it down:

- Must be over 50 – am not spilling my guts to any snowflakes.

- Must have lots of letters after their name – don't want someone who just did a 2-hour course on a Saturday afternoon at the local tech analysing me.

- Must look quite wide awake (Joan at work went to a therapist and was raging when she realised the therapist wasn't reflecting on her poignant musings but had fallen asleep halfway through the session. To be really fair I often feel the eyelids drooping when Joan starts banging on but for £75 an hour I'd make more of an effort).

I then look through the pictures. In one the therapists is wearing a jumper with bows and kittens. Seriously? I instantly rule her out. And the one with hair pretty much covering her face. And the one that looks suspiciously like a serial killer. And the one that has a very very low cut top on – like so low cut I still wonder if she had another career and got the photos mixed up. And the names – I can't go to a therapist called Poppy. I just can't.

Then I have a panic – what if there is a Loony List somewhere – and I end up on it due to something I say in the sessions. I Google again. Apparently the only time a therapist breaks total confidentiality is if the patient says something that may cause them to be a danger to themselves or others. I resolve not to mention the many times I consider banging my partner over the head with our heaviest frying pan. Or the notion I have sometimes to take to bed for a year with just boxes of Galaxy for sustenance.

Finally I find someone who seems to be relatively sane and sorted – Tracey Winfrey. I buy Psychologies magazine and have a good read as I want to appear knowledgeable and as if I do this all the time when I rock up. I also treat myself to some glittery sketchers as it seems appropriate.

When I get there I am thinking that maybe I shouldn't have gone. I am not a Fruit Loop. I am perfectly OK and normal. I might be ay OK without the HRT. I might not resort back to screaming at people who drop litter or don't pick up dog shit/telling various people at work to eff off/crying at Save the Donkey campaigns and giving them all my money. Maybe that was just a little blip in my otherwise sane and sorted life.

I get in and the therapist gives me a big form to read over and sign. She is talking about data protection and other stuff that goes a bit over my head as I am not really listening as I am thinking more and more this was a mistake. There is an open box of tissues and I look at them knowing I won't need them as I only cry when it is totally inappropriate and unnecessary. I have forgotten my glasses and for some reason don't want to say – so do a passible impression of reading the form and sign it with a flourish. Then I am slightly anxious that I have just signed up to 50 sessions and will have to remortgage my house to pay.

She doesn't say 'umm' and 'ahh' like Suzie did… she blethers on for a bit and I am starting to get a bit bored and am digging my nails into my hand to stay awake. I am feeling a fraud tbh – she probably deals with people with serious addictions like alcohol and drugs and here I am trying to quit the galaxy counters. I am wanting to tell her that I need her to stop me telling people to feck off; bursting into tears for no reason; and wanting to stay in bed all day a lot. But then she says something – and I don't know what. But I am talking… and talking… and talking… and talking. And by the end of the session I feel I have diagnosed and cured myself. I sit back very proud of myself – waiting for her to issue me a refund and say no point in coming back.

"Hmm Let me just reflect back some of the things you have said" she muses – and starts to say things. That apparently I have said. But she must be making them up to drum up more business – surely I did not say such things. But they do sound a little familiar.

So I think I may go back – she doesn't have glittery shoes – but they aren't quite the deal breaker I thought!

CHAPTER 43

Things not to say to a menopausal woman

In this chapter, I bring to you – my meno-musings on the top 20 things to never say to a menopausal woman.

1. I just sailed through it no problems at all

2. I have heard it can take about 15 years to go through it

3. Have you forgotten your HRT today hahahaha

4. Are you taking part in Movember?

5. We have run out of chocolate

6. Ohh I didn't want to say as I wasn't sure – but you are aren't you... you're pregnant! Imagine – at your age – what a lovely bump!

7. Don't you think you are maybe overreacting

8. Let's put the heating up a bit

9. It could be all in your head – after all ____ and ____ didn't have any problems at all

10. We have run out of wine

11. There is something stuck to your chin – a hair or something... oh um – it seems to be attached... umm... oh sorry

12. Calm down!

13. Nice whiskers!

14. Wow! You have gained wei... umm I mean – wow, you look well

15. Let's go out and stay up 'til 3am

16. It can't be that bad!

17. Let's go to bed – not to sleep – but to shag all night

18. My Granny is going through it too – you are just like her

19. We seem to have no alcohol in the house

20. Check out what Gwyneth Paltrow is saying about it all.

CHAPTER 44

To Santa, love from menopausal me

In this chapter, I bring to you – my meno-musings in writing my letter to Santa.

Dear Santa

I think at this point you may be sitting checking your list – even checking it twice. (I hope you have noted the recent data protection regulations changes in making your list up – we are being bored shitless at work about it so feels unfair if you are escaping it)

Anyway – it's been 40 years since I wrote to you – I still haven't quite forgiven you for that bloody pink bike with a flowery bell when I EXPLICITLY asked for a BMX bike. But I am willing to let that go. Anyone can make a mistake. Which leads me onto this 'naughty or nice' thing you talk of.

I would like a bit of clarity on exactly what you mean by nice? And also if you would consider hormones a reasonable mitigating circumstance.

So I accept my regular thoughts on bashing my partner on the head with a frying pan aren't exactly 'nice' but I didn't ever actually do it! So I don't think that is enough justification for a place on the naughty list. And yes I know gluttony is a sin – and I have had way, way too much chocolate and pizza this year. Yes, I have canceled a number of plans at the last minute when I realised I'd have to actually leave the house and pretended to be ill so that I can just watch Netflix. I know that's not great but I'm telling you – if you suffered menopausal exhaustion you'd struggle even though you only work one day a year. And yes I accidentally-on-purpose spilled my hot coffee on a guy who annoyed me. But tbh – he was a bit of a tosser and played his bloody music without headphones at 7am. I have had a number of honesty moments especially with the snowflake generation which on reflection silence would have been better – but don't you think that maybe it is my gift to the next generation.

Anyway here is my list:

- A libido

- A flat stomach
- A non-hairy chin
- A Jo Malone candle (not one of those replacements from TK Maxx – they are not the same)
- A self-cleaning house
- Legislation declaring six months fully paid menopausal leave
- A pension
- An alibi for when I murder Alan at work.

To be honest, I will probably have forgotten this list by Christmas. Well, not the slim tummy and libido. Don't forget them.

CHAPTER 45

Trying to be organised

In this chapter, I bring to you – my musings on trying to be an organised woman on Christmas Eve.

So the day in question started fairly ok. I had to get up at 3am and have a shower due to either hot flush or the flu. Am not sure which. But then I went back to sleep and slept solidly 'til 9am. I felt most smug when I got up as I have Christmas sorted this year. One of the few benefits I am finding of the menopause is that less and less fucks are given as time goes on. So instead of weeks of prep I ordered a massive steak pie from the butcher and bought frozen roast potatoes and frozen parsnips from Tesco. I then asked all my guests to bring between them a starter, a pudding, cheese and biscuits – and all their own booze. Done!! I can now laze about all day. Aided by my lovely dog walking friend who has no dogs of her own and so wants to come and take Sweet Dog up a Munro – double hooray.

Following on with my natural approach to my menopause symptoms, I mix a soya yoghurt with an egg and chia seeds and some porridge oats and frozen fruit and pop it all in the oven for 40 minutes. I am a bit fluey and I spy a little tiny bottle of whisky. I mix it into a cup with lemon and some honey – blitz it in microwave and head through to watch some telly while my breakfast gets ready. I feel quite proud of my 'no stress' Christmas, Get me at 20 minutes to 11am drinking whisky with nothing to do!

20 to 11... 20 to 11... FUCK... FUCKITY FUCK... The bastarding steak pie that I ordered last week. The butcher warned me that I MUST get it by 11am or he will be closed. He called me yesterday to remind me. I forget everything so I put it on a Post-it on the kettle. But I didn't have tea did I... No, I had to have bloody whisky.

I drag on some jogging trousers, tuck my nightie in, pull on my trainers and grab the car keys. Oh no – the bloody whisky!! Am I over the limit? Can't risk it. Grab Sweet Dog as she needs a walk and may as well kill two birds with one stone and tear out the house. Tear back two mins later to turn off oven containing my lovely healthy breakfast. Tear back out again. Five minutes into fast walk/slow jog Sweet Dog starts to ominously start the twirling that always ends in a massive shit. And FUCK I have no poo bags.

None – I forgot to lift them. A fellow dog walker takes sympathy and gives me two – just in case. I almost cry with gratitude, scoop up the massive shit and toss it in the bin and keep running. I have to get to the butcher or we have no Christmas main course. I try not to berate myself as the mindfulness part of my menopause book says to be kind to yourself. But for God's sake – I had ONE BLOODY JOB!!

I get there at 2 mins past 11 – and thank God there are two people in front of me. I take a breath and realise I have forgotten my phone... And remember the dog walking lady... NO NO NO – I cannot miss her – I'd forgotten she was coming. I need Sweet Dog tired out. And now I can't phone her.

The butcher's daughter comes out with a tub of Celebrations – chocolate is good. And she is only 11 and doesn't say anything or judge when I take 4. I go to pop one in my mouth and smell something horrible. It is dog poo... on my nail. The rushed scooping lead to a smear of shit – on ME! I wipe it on my jogging trousers and scoff the chocolates. I get my steak pie and head off at a run to try and get back for Dog Walking Lady.

But Sweet Dog can smell the steak pie. Sweet Dog wants steak pie. Sweet Dog jumps up and adds muddy dog prints to her shit stains onto my trousers. Sweet Dog continues in this manner all the way home. She is nothing if not persistent. Resist urge to kick bloody Sweet Dog. It is pissing down and me, Sweet Dog and pie are all getting soaked.

We get back. I strip my shit covered soaking wet paw stained trousers and all the rest of my clothes and fling them in the washing machine – chuck in the bold and turn it on. My healthy breakfast is all disgustingly half cooked and cold so I chuck it out. Fuck it – I am having what I had planned for Christmas breakfast tomorrow – my favourite – morning roll with thick butter, tomato ketchup, Lorne sausage and a potato scone. I stick the sausage in the oven – bit healthier if I grill rather than fry it – and fling some chia seeds on the butter in the roll. I need to at least make an effort. I run upstairs – quick shower and dressing gown on – then tank back down for my breakfast.

There is an ominous clunk clunk coming from the washing machine. FUCK – it is my fanny magnet. My £35 fanny magnet. Not even 48 hours old. In the washing machine. I frantically Google to find out if it is still effective after such an ordeal. But of course, this is related to the menopause so answers to such sensible questions are not to be found.

Give up and retreat to the TV to watch the Bette Davies and Joan Crawford feud that I recorded from last night (there are two women who were defo menopausal during Baby Jane!) with my amazing breakfast which does cheer me up.

In all the stuff I have read about symptoms of the menopause, 'memory lapses and fuzzy thinking' appear as a simple bullet point. This post is just one tiny example of what that little bullet point means in real life!!!

Christmas Eve starts at last. The advice is that alcohol is not good for menopausal women.

I beg to feckin differ!!!

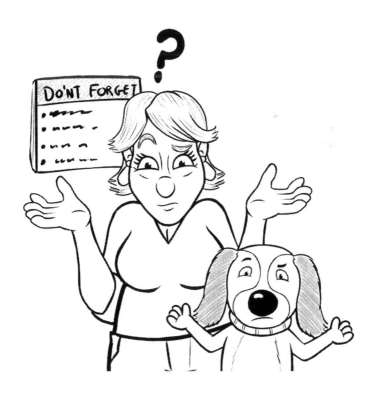

CHAPTER 46

The fuckit bucket

My fucks are disappearing in direct correlation to the disappearance of my memory, eggs, eyebrows, waist and wrinkle-free skin.

But the loss of fucks I find something to celebrate. I gave so many fucks when I was younger. Far too many fucks – but now they are flying into my metaphorical Fuck Bucket – which is fit to overflow now. I look back fondly sometimes at those fucks but in the same way as I look fondly back at my pink legwarmers and sequinned boob tubes. With no desire to resurrect them but with an understanding that I was young and daft then.

The Fucks I used to give if people didn't like me – gone! As I now realise that people will like me or not like me – and most of the time it will be nothing at all to do with me.

Fucks about giving my opinion. Gone. I'd rather be hated for being me than liked for pretending to be someone else. I spent years worrying what people thought of me – then I stopped worrying about it. Now I realise no-one was really thinking about me as much as I was thinking they did!

No fucks about buying the latest most expensive cosmetics Coz no-one no one is looking at my eyes and thinking 'maybe that mascara is Sisley or maybe it's Maybelline'.

Zero fucks about getting 'bikini body ready' and zero fucks about the fashion stylists saying a one piece is more flattering for the 'older' woman. Fuck that – my pink bikini goes on and voila – there is my bikini body ready to go! I give zero fucks about magazines that aim to bring women down and treat them like second class citizens unless they portray what they believe a woman should look like (I mean wtf with these eyebrows that start at the tear duct and end at the lug!).

I look back on my life and realise it was the fucks I didn't give that enhanced my life. The fucks I didn't give about packing my job in and travelling... the fucks I didn't give about toxic people I eliminated from my life... I could go on and on. But in conclusion – freedom truly is another word for very few fucks left to give. I'm through with self-doubt and 'playing nice'.

And I do have a few fucks left – but I spend them wisely now. And the power of a Fuck consciously directed by a menopausal women should not be underestimated. The Charity that continually harassed my elderly neighbour when his wife died with phone calls and letters asking for more and more money which he, feeling vulnerable, was giving although he was living on a tiny pension (this harassment apparently due to the fact he'd done a collection for them in her memory at the funeral!). I gave a huge fuck about that. I mean a MASSIVE fuck. That fuck is probably still reverberating round that charities office now.

One benefit of getting older is that you realise that freedom is just another word for very few fucks left to give. And we find ourselves unfuckwithable due their disappearance!

Anyone else chucking more and more fucks into the fuck bucket?

CHAPTER 47

CELEBRATING 50ths

In this chapter, I bring to you – my meno-musings on the 50th Birthday celebrations.

I mused on this during a weekend spent in the Lakes celebrating Tina the Turners birthday – the second in a slew of 50s happening over this year.

Tina the Turner isn't actually 50 'til October but she decreed long ago that any birthday she had that that finished with a 0 must last a full year. And who are we to differ?

This one was special as the last time we were all together (due to Geography and Life) was for her 21st. Even with menopausal brain fog, it didn't take long to work out that was 29 years ago. 'How can this be?' we mused, convinced that we surely cannot have been on this planet long enough to have lived almost 3 decades since we were 21. We certainly do not have the wisdom one would expect from such life experience and thanks to L'Oréal we have no grey hairs either! Further analysis concluded that most of us are now in our sixth decade on this planet. FuckaDuck!

Travel arrangements were complex with no-one wanting to travel in my car due to my tendency to roll the windows down during a hot flush. Often this isn't a huge problem, but I guess this reluctance is currently understandable as it is currently minus 8 with frequent blizzards. However, the other options for the non-drivers were Pee Stop Pam who has to pull into every service station to go and have a wee, and Easily Distracted Rachel whose driving since hitting the menopause has become erratic to say the least. So I got my lovely pal Rosie and we compromised that I would roll the window down only twice, and she would keep a rug in the footwell to use at these times. A sensible solution for two sensible adults. I remember for the 21st we were only bothered about how much booze we could ram into the car – how times change!

And so Six menopausal women went off to the Lakes. We were joined by Tina's 35-year-old cousin, Jane who lives near our cottage. She is quite funky and set us all up a WhatsApp group. We got to our location to discover she had posted a number of bars and pubs in Penrith and found a taxi firm that could take us there.

How we laughed!!! We were still laughing at half seven when she arrived to find us putting on our pyjamas. We chat about the best slippers to wear to keep warm. I favour a stout all enclosed fur lined slipper but Tina is on other end of the spectrum – not quite ready to give up her mules. Slipper socks seemed the most popular. Jane tries not to let her disappointment show at our mirth at the thought of actually getting dressed up and going out somewhere.

We all then poured the gin and started a game of Cards against Humanity. I had never heard of this and having now played several rounds – I can state with some authority that this is not a game to play if you or any of your friends are easily offended. Fortunately this did not apply to any of us. However we had to scrap all the cards that required two answers as Kerry was getting pissed off with most of us forgetting the start of the question before we got to the end. Her time will come!!!

Then we had a nice long chat about all the illnesses we have suffered from over the year. I learned more about the human anatomy that most GP's that night. Then we moved onto the importance of having a will and how expensive a funeral can be. Finally we moved onto pensions which was depressing as we all thought we had an agreement with the Government that we would work our arses off from the age of 16 and give the Government lots of our income in order to get a wee bit back from the age of 60. However the government broke their side of the bargain by using our cash to pay for failed IT systems, bombs and Duck Ponds for MP's. Hence we will all be working 'til we are around 145 years old. We were so depressed at that thought we had to have another gin before we sorted out all our rubbish for the recycling bins the next day.

Menopausal memory loss and no Facebook in those days' means we have only a hazy recollection of the 21st – but I think I can categorically state we did not discuss pensions or do any recycling...

Next day we decide to hit the spa. I have a slight problem in that I always assumed swimsuits fell into the same category as earrings, shoes and handbags i.e useable however fat you get. Well turns out that is not the case. It took some serious wrestling to get it over my hips and especially my belly – then it clung like a sausage skin about to split at any time.

Fortunately there were lovely big baggy robes for us to enjoy. Didn't stop me having four cakes, two scones and seven sandwiches with prosecco for high tea though (another change from the 21st – everyone scoffed everything in those days – I have not changed but many of my pals now following diets to help their symptoms. Carb free... Vegan... Vegetarian. This means lots of extra for me who follows no such diet except for occasional fad ones.

We then had to head back to the lodge as a camomile tea and a disco nap is essential when attempting to party two nights in a row.

There seemed no point in taking our pyjamas off after the disco nap so we all came together to sing karaoke and drink more gin. Disaster struck when we ran out of mixers!! However Tina had the great idea of using prosecco instead of tonic water. It was a great idea – rhubarb and ginger gin topped up with prosecco is very good. We then experimented with other 'mixers' such as Pina colada vodka. Things got a little messy from there on in. Let's just say a good night was had by all. And as we are all technologically inept there is no evidence on Instagram, Pinterest, Snapchat, Twitter or any of the other things that the yoof of today use. We did do a couple of photos for Facebook which according to Kerry is just for old people but they were very much 'before' pictures as none of us could work the camera or video after a few.

Next morning it was off home – so we all had just half a cup of tea each so we wouldn't have to do a toilet stop until we had been driving for at least an hour. We are nothing if not sensible. We then got all the bananas, grapes, vegetables that we had optimistically brought and watched go mushy over the weekend and took them to the recycling bins along with the 20 billion empty bottles and 60 billion empty cake crisps and dips and sweet wrappers

Happy Birthday 50-year-olds everywhere! If it is true that things get better with age then we are all MAGNIFICENT!

CHAPTER 48

Juicing

In this chapter, I bring to you – my meno-musings on juicing.

I am sure this will work in my battle of the bulge.

I had done the tit/tum test (where success is walking towards a wall and having your tits hit the wall before your tum does) and failed miserably.

I knew things had got really bad when I was watching a news item on obesity. You know the ones – always accompanied by video footage of shoulder to knee views of poor unsuspecting Fat Bastards going about their business. And I suddenly became filled with terror that I was about to come into view – wandering down Princes Street eating a roll and sausage or a burger or something similar with the camera zooming in on my jelly belly and everyone watching saying 'oh that looks like Jen... wait a minute... that IS her'. That night I dreamed of post after post on my Facebook saying 'saw you on the news last night' with a freeze frame of my jelly belly – then a ton of comments from Daily Mail readers slagging me off for single-handedly bringing the NHS to its knees. I woke with palpitations and thanks to Google can confirm this is most likely to be another menopausal symptom rather than a heart attack which I first thought.

So it was time to take action. I prepared for the scales in the usual way – no breakfast; trip to loo beforehand; gave a pint of blood the day before etc.

Deep breath – it would be small step for a skinny woman – but it is a giant leap for a fat menopausal woman.

Pause. Look down.

Oh...

My...

God!!!

Officially 50% fatter than I was 8 years ago. About 40% of that increase resting around my middle.

And it is 12 weeks 'til I attend another wedding. A wedding where a number of people won't have seen me for eight years. I need to lose 70lbs by then. This is a challenge in itself – but will be made more challenging due to a large number of 50th Birthdays between now and then.

Now, Davina McCall spent her 50th with her friends – trekking about 600 miles with only a tiny slice of vegan cake half way to sustain them. I tentatively suggested similar activities to my almost 50-year-old friends only to be met with great mirth and a reminder to pay my share of the five-course tasting menus with cocktails/ weekend away with full breakfast and three-course dinner... and other such celebrations all equally unlikely to support 'Project Lose 70'.

I will not be put off though. I will not give in to menopausal fatness. I will fight fight fight for the return of my body to its rightful shape.

So I decide to juice. Easy Peasy. Amanda Holden does it – she did an interview and it was accompanied by her photo in tight workout gear clutching her green drink and looking fab. And my menopause book says that increasing my intake of live, fresh fruits and vegetables will help my body 'eat its way out of menopausal symptoms'. And the blurb says I can lose 5lbs in 7 days which the biggest motivator.

Got my juicer out the attic (I did it once about a year ago but it took bloody ages to clean it so I didn't use it again – but I am more determined this time) and go to Tesco and buy an inordinate amount of fruit and veg.

And I actually did it – following it completely (apart from four freddo frogs, a marmalade sandwich and a packet of love hearts... but I bet even Amanda Holden didn't stick to it 100%).

Four day big weigh-in this morning. And... I LOST 6LB! I dance around with Sweet Dog, much to her joy.

I am losing more than average... it suddenly strikes me that perhaps I don't have a metabolism shot to pieces from the menopause but am actually just a greedy bastard...

Another 64lbs to go. Well, 54lbs as I am going to get a fake tan before the wedding and everyone knows a tan knocks 10lbs off! Actually maybe 44lbs because careful dressing can knock another 10lbs off according to Trinnie and Susannah.

Project Lose 44 is now well underway.

CHAPTER 49

Back to work

In this chapter, I bring to you – my meno-musings on going back to work with the best of intentions.

My plan when I returned from work after a break was to pick out outfits for each day, iron them and choose matching shoes and accessories.

Before you think 'what a saddo' – the reason is that being menopausal over the Christmas holidays is one thing (lying in bed 'til noon with Catch Up telly and a never-ending supply of rum and chocolate then enjoying shopping and lunching with friends will ease even the worst menopausal symptoms). But being menopausal and having to work is quite another. And one of my resolutions is to get rid of the morning 'before work' stress and get each day off to as good a start as possible. I also went into work one day last year with odd shoes on so want to avoid that if I can.

I do think menopausal leave should be debated in parliament. There is maternity leave, carers leave, parental leave and God knows what kind of leave so why not menopausal leave? This would be done on a case by case basis – so all the feckers that declare they 'sailed through' their menopause and 'barely noticed 'til it was over' get no leave at all – it gets added to people like me who are finding it somewhat more of a challenge. And in fact those who do 'sail through' should be made to work twice as many hours and clean nightclub toilets at the weekends and maybe pick up dog poo for people out walking their dogs 'til the smug look drops from their bloody faces.

Anyway – I digress – back to New Me! I was also going to start healthy eating today – with a breakfast of oats and fresh fruit and then later make up a delicious packed lunch for work with flax seeds, berries and nuts and many things that are recommended to assist you to cope with the menopause.

However, things did not really go to plan. I had maybe one or nine glasses of wine too many last night and many friends stayed over. So this morning I had to have two bacon rolls with quite a bit of butter and tomato sauce as it isn't really fair to impose my healthy eating habits onto other people.

I then decided it would be just as well to open and finish off the last box of Thornton's as if they were in the house they would just cause temptation when I start 'for real' tomorrow.

I did try and pick outfits for work but this ended up in a lot of cursing and swearing as it would appear pretty much all my work clothes have shrunk while I have been off. A clamber into the attic then ensued to find my bag of 'fattest ever clothes' which also proved a tad tight and smelt a bit funny so had to wash all of them and stretch them while drying so I can go to work tomorrow in something other than my pyjamas (which are still fitting great). I was always against elasticated waists in all but pyjamas but my expanding girth is putting in repeated requests for such a feature.

I was then sweaty and thirsty and fed up and the thought of wearing leggings and smocks 'til my arse and belly shrink a bit is a trifle depressing. So I'm afraid to admit that I have fallen at the first fence of alcohol-free lifestyle that I had planned – with a lovely bottle of white which is going down well with the left-over Doritos and cheese and chive dip from last night. The books say alcohol is not good for the menopause and maybe it isn't but I can say with complete certainty that it helps you give less of a fuck about it.

Meeting after meeting with a hangover at work is not very good though. I remember in my 20s desperately wanting to be invited to meetings. Then in my 30s I felt great when I was invited to meetings – I was important! Now I will do anything to avoid bloody meetings.

One of my lovely friends who 'found the menopause so liberating and a time of great energy' told me that she found a sense of spirituality and connectedness as she went through her 'journey' (it's not the bloody X factor I felt like saying but I didn't as I can't risk losing any more friends due to menopausal grumpiness). I have been a bit adrift over the last few months though – and wondering about things like mindfulness courses or maybe retraining to be a dog groomer or packing everything in to travel round Greece for a year or maybe setting up a social enterprise Café. I have started a number of things that never ever get finished despite initial flushes of enthusiasm.

So I am looking deep into myself. I am reading self-help guides that tell me I must banish consumerism'. Really? It is clear the author has not yet been to the Joules or White Stuff sale this year or they may have reworded that part! (Paperchase is worth a look too). And I must also apparently stop gossiping. I beg to differ! I think we can guarantee the author did not consult with menopausal women on this message – waves of empty chatter along with a bit of retail therapy is what keeps us (well me anyway) going. Maybe next year I will get round to writing a self-help book for menopausal women.

I think I've just found my direction and purpose!! And right after I've finished my chocolates, wine and Doritos and watched another box set – I will get going on it.

CHAPTER 50

Advice for the menopausal woman's significant others

In this chapter, I bring to you – my meno-musings on advice for the menopausal woman's significant others.

Or to be more specific – for the HABPSO's (Husbands and Boyfriends and Partners and Significant Others) of menopausal women.

I get tons of messages from women saying their HABPSO's just don't 'get' the menopause and are being less than supportive!

So I thought I'd take things a step further and dedicate a whole post to the people supporting a women through their menopausal years.

One thing that can help is to live 24 hours as a menopausal woman – this immersion will give you real insight into what it's like and allow you to empathise more fully.

So this is how to have such a day:

- Start the experiment about 10pm – go to bed with a thermal vest, four jumpers with hot water bottles between each – and keep your electric blanket on full.

- Once you are soaked through with sweat, get up and change the bedclothes and yourself.

- Ensure you have a recording of all the things you are worried about. Set your alarm for 3am and listen to it for 2 hours.

- Just before you are about to fall asleep again – stick a bag of midgies or mosquitos in bed with you and lie itching and scratching for an hour or so.

- Get up and wear clothes that are a size too small around the waist.

- Before going to work tweeze your beard rather than shave.

- Smoke 5 joints and take 2 sleeping tablets and a swig of Night Nurse on your way to work. This will get you some way to understanding the 'brain fog' symptom.

- Every couple of hours (ideally before a key meeting with your boss) get up and nip to the kitchen and stand in front of the industrial-sized ovens for a full 10 minutes. * Halfway through meetings think of something very very sad and try to hold back the tears. If someone annoys you tell them to shut up and then worry about it for the rest of the day.

- That evening allow your partner to rub your 'joystick' with coarse sandpaper for a long time.

This will help you get a full understanding of what the woman in your life is going through. If this isn't sufficient to get you to modify your behaviour around her – here are some really specific tips:

- If you arrive home and find said lady completely naked on top of the bed – DO NOT and I repeat DO NOT take this as an invitation to leap on her for some passion. The correct response is to say 'hunni are you a bit hot – let me just get you some cold wine out of the fridge'.

- There are times when the lovely lady may tell you to 'get to fuck and when you get there just keep fucking off and fucking off 'til you have fucked right off'. If this happens think very carefully if this is justified – perhaps you have maybe been breathing just a bit too loudly? Or returned from Marks and Spencer having picked up the cheese rather than the chocolate profiteroles for the dessert option, or worse the alcohol-free option over the wine option, from the Dine In offer? The correct response is 'Oh darling let me get you some wine and I'll sleep in the spare room so you get some space'.

- You may face a situation where you see some whiskers clearly visible on the ladies chin or upper lip. And you wonder whether to ask if she is taking part in Movember. Don't. Just don't. Just give her some wine.

- You may find your lovely partner tells you the same thing seven or eight or even fourteen times. It is not recommended to say "U have told me that already" or to interrupt and say "yes I KNOW" ...instead, just pretend it's the first time you heard it and consider it practice for when the Alzheimer's kicks in.

- Some nights you may notice the woman sticking a leg in then out of the covers then in then out again. It is not the correct response to sing the hokey cokey at full volume. This isn't even vaguely funny. Not even a little bit.

- You may be woken several times in the night with the woman suffering anxiety and wanting to talk about whether Joan Parks at work meant anything when she looked at her funny last week. The correct response is NOT 'oh don't be stupid and let me bloody sleep'. You must say 'let me get some wine and you can tell me all about it'. Even if she has already told you 18 times and forgotten about it.

- A particularly dangerous scenario is when your other half asks 'do I look fat in this?' I would hope no advice is needed here. But just in case – the correct answer is NOT 'yes you do a bit' or 'you'll do'. You must look up from your phone and say 'WOW you look AMAZING, let me get you some wine'.

I hope this helps all you HABPSO's. Menopausal women... feel free to print it and staple it to your HABPSO"s forehead if you feel they need to focus a bit more.

CHAPTER 51

Let's all do Movember

In this chapter, I bring to you – my meno-musings on Movember and why we should maybe all join the men for this one.

I mused on this when Movember was almost upon us. An annual event involving the men of the world growing moustaches during the month of November to raise awareness of men's health issues.

The guys at work were all chatting about it yesterday with some deciding they would take it a step further and do a beard too. A competition was then set up where the winner would be the most hairy face on the 30th November.

"I think I'll join you," I said as a joke. But no one laughed. This was a bit worrying – it could be because I work with nerdy geeks who genuinely have not actually realised I am a woman. But it might also be because they see it as a viable option for me. Menopausal paranoia hits – maybe even they are worried I will win the competition over their bum fluff chins. Because I am sure if I left my face to its own devices I would win hands down.

My bathroom has bright lights and a magnifying mirror facing the window and several pairs of superstrong tweezers to fight the battle of the stubble. There are tweezers in the car and in all my handbags. If I am ever on desert island discs I'd have to lie and say something high brow like 'I'd take 'crime and punishment' with me to read as my luxury item' – but the reality it would be tweezers. The battle against the bristle gets tougher every day!

Indeed maybe all women should participate in Movember – I would be interested to know just how hairy I can get without daily intervention. Women of a certain age could do it to raise awareness of the menopause. Maybe I am onto something here. It could perhaps lead to another career. Like the singing bearded lady in 'The Greatest Showman'. Except I can't sing. Or I could at least get equal pay for this career by masquerading as a man!

But they are but fantasies – the reality is very different. I woke up at 3am the other day paralysed with fear that I might end up in a coma and would end up with a massive beard and moustache and visitors to my bedside would laugh at me. This is what happens when menopausal anxiety and menopausal sleeplessness collide! I checked with Google to see if hair still grew when you were in a coma – and apparently it does. So I woke my partner up to get them to promise on Sweet Dog's life that they would attend to my beard and moustache if ever such a fate befell me. Initially the response was 'oh for fucks sake' followed by what I think was an attempt at dark humour "I would just pull the bloody plug" but after a wee chat there was more understanding (well it was more 'if I bloody agree to this will you shut up and let me sleep' than full understanding but it was sufficient to reassure me).

I have tried electrolysis – but it is not as Chantelle the therapist told me 'like someone gently flicking your skin' it was more like 'someone stabbing you with a red-hot needle loads and loads of times. It cost £90 (which is about three bottles of Jack Daniels and a bottle of Pinot) and made not one iota of difference!

I tried waxing but then had to walk about for days with a red rash all over my face that resembled shaving rash or the plague depending on the light. And, like threading (which was so sore it made me cry), that was after having to hide away for a week while the hairs grew to a suitable length to wax/thread. So neither could be classed as an overall success.

My mum recommended hair lightener but I am not sure a blonde beard and moustache would be much more flattering than a dark one.

Hmmm – I have a plan!! I am going to suggest that on the 1st December they all have the beards/moustaches removed using waxing/threading/electrolysis – in public to raise money for a Men's Health Charity.

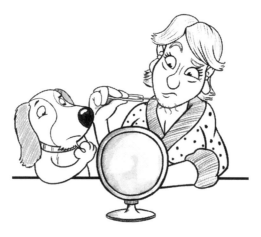

CHAPTER 52

Giving up on Fat Class

In this chapter, I bring to you my musings of telling the Fat Class to Feck off and just keep fecking off 'til it has fecked right off!

My musings started on the day I was due to go back to Fat Class today after missing it for a couple of weeks on account of being a Fatso who had gained weight for the second week in a row and was too mortified to make it three weeks on a row.

And I thought it would be a hugely successful visit with lots of clapping for me and getting to share my story of all the exciting Quark recipes I had used while everyone looked at me with envy at my amazing weight loss. This vision was not because of the huge amounts of Quark, yoghurt in my cupboard and packs of steak in the fridge and tons and tons of fruit and veg everywhere. Not because I stuck to the plan (I mean – God who does do that for a full week?). But because I have had flu. And have barely eaten a thing. I started with an upset stomach and I thought maybe one of the new menopause supplements I was trying. But nope – next day on fire, throat hurting, head hurting, bones hurting. Resulting in three days in bed with no meals. So I had predicted a massive weight loss.

Then I had a wee pre-weight in – and was raging!!! I weigh the exact same as when I started – ie I have regained the entire half stone I lost. FFS!!!! How can that be? I am a freak of feckin nature. I was ranting and jumping naked on and off the scales so it was very brave of my partner to come and see what they could do to help.

I was emotional anyway even before realising I was once again a Fatty. Declining estrogen puts you in a permanent state of PMS. So when pre-menstrual it is a double whammy. I had to pull over before I crashed the car earlier in the day as Ed Sheeran's Supermarket Flowers came on and I sobbed and sobbed and couldn't see the road or control the steering wheel. Then someone at work asked if I had any kids and when I said No they said 'oh what a shame – did it just not happen for you?' I am so over this shite – I do not need or want sympathy for being childless. I used to nod and say 'yes oh well aren't you lucky to have kids' etc and try and hide the boredom as they told me about their offspring. But the 'Don't Give a Fuck' hormones had taken over. She rambled on with smug smiles, 'I have three – I just can't imagine life without them. I don't think it would be worth living '. I interrupted her "What a shame!'. She was most shocked 'What? she gasped'. 'Yes I said it must be awful to have three children and absolutely no life without them' I said. She wasn't smiling now. But I was on a roll. 'The tiredness. The cost. The sheer tedium. I don't know how you do it? My life would not be worth living if I had three kids. I am so glad I dodged that bullet'. My quite nice work colleague Jane said later I had maybe gone too far. But to be honest I was just getting warmed up – I managed to offend quite a few others by the end of the day. The thing with hormonal rage is that you just don't know if you are hormonal or if the person you are dealing with is just a twat. Today I think I was mainly justified. I am just going to check our disciplinary process though just to see if declining estrogen is a mitigating circumstance... just to be sure.

Anyway, I digress – again. Back to bloody gaining weight when not even eating. My partner must have been feeling brave. 'You did have lots of those honey throat lozenges – and all that cough syrup and Lemsips'. 'THAT'S MEDICINE' I screeched. 'IT DOESN'T COUNT'. 'I think it does' was the mild reply. I looked it up – feck – it is true – throat lozenges – one and a half naughty points each and I was necking about 20 a day. Lemsips – half a naughty point each and I was drinking them one after the other – each with a massive shot of honey and a whisky in the evening one.

'Remember as well you were having cans of coke coz you said the bubbles helped by scratching your throat' my partner helpfully continued. Shit – yes I had forgotten about that – 7 naughty points a can and I had about 3 a day. 'And remember when we got the dine in for a tenner deal?' My partner continued perhaps not realising that I was about to do a menopausal equivalent of the Incredible Hulk as I was being made very angry by all these reminders...

'You ate it all – the full chicken and the veg and the wine – I was too ill' I snapped. 'Yes but you said you would eat all the chocolate profiteroles as the cold cream inside them would help your throat. I suggested you eat some of the feckin tubs of Quark that are in the fridge but you said they tasted like shit'. This is true – I had forgotten about that. And I suddenly remembered eating a tub of Ben and Jerry's for a similar reason while I was alone watching loose women from my bed. I decided not to vocalise that – my partner was having too much bloody fun without adding that in. 'And remember your mum brought you a box of chocolates to cheer you up'.

'I beg to feckin differ – we SHARED those' I snapped. 'Well no' said my partner who is just a bit too feckin literal at the moment –

'you gave me the coffee one and the nut one because you didn't like them – but you scoffed the rest – even the strawberry one and you know that is my favourite'.

So it would appear that perhaps gaining weight is not so surprising but ffs I have been POORLY. It wouldn't be so bad if I had been out getting bevvied having fun and scoffing three-course meals. But seems totally crap that all the medicinal things have made me a chubster again.

So I am not going back to Fat Class. I don't think it was really me. Almost 100 quid on the pass and the books and the shite Fat Lass bars and stressing and worrying and chopping and cooking – just to end up where I started. And a night a week happy clapping and talking about how to make chocolate out of bran flakes or empty toilet rolls with a spoon of cocoa powder or whatever it was. Life is just too short for that bollocks. My decision confirmed by my pal who is re-joining as she stated 'it is the only thing that works'. She has been starting and restarting for five years and is 2 stone heavier than when she first started. Isn't that is the definition of madness – doing the same thing but expecting a different result?

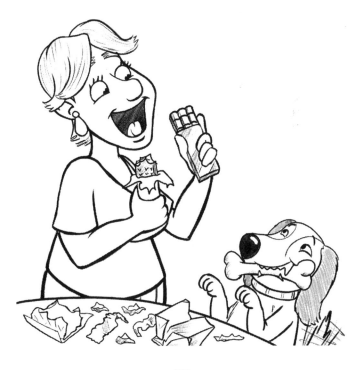

CHAPTER 53

12 Days of Christmas

In this chapter, I bring to you – my musings on what my true love brought to me!

On the 12th day of Christmas my true love sent to me...

12 Incontinence pads

11 Different moods a day

10 Wiry chin Hairs

9 Episodes of brain fog

8 Hot flushes

7 Aching joints

6 Missed periods

5 Pairs of comfy sketchers

4 Missed periods

3 Just in case tampons

2 Hours sleep a night

And a bladder that is very very LEAKEYYYYYYY!

CHAPTER 54

Having a Fuck It! list

In this chapter, I bring to you my most important meno-musings – the importance of having a Fuck It! list

Going through the menopause is a bit shit but it is better than the alternative!! Without being too maudlin – getting to an age where you experience it is a privilege denied to many.

So I have decided to celebrate instead of having my usual whinge. I have developed a Fuck it! list.

Everyone has heard of a Bucket List – things to do before you die. Usually quite big things like jumping out of a plane over the Grand Canyon. Or hiking up Machu Picchu. Or volunteering to count frogs in Costa Rica.

But a 'Fuck it!' list doesn't have to be anything major – just things you always fancied doing but kept putting off without really being sure why. It can't be things like losing weight or drinking hot water with lemon every morning or anything like that. The test is to put Fuck it before the thing you are going to do – eg You wouldn't say 'Fuck it I am going to eat 1000 calories a day and drink 2 litres of water for three months'. But you might say 'Fuck it I'm getting my belly button pierced'

So now – with more of the runway of life behind me than in front of me – has there ever been a better time to say Fuck It? To face people who sneer – and say I'm going to do it anyway!

My first 'Fuck It' came when I went to get a new car. I am a sensible driver – always had a wee car – cheap for petrol, low tax, low insurance. But I was passing a showroom – and a bright purple sports car was in the forecourt. I went in. Two-litre engine. Leather Seats. Purple... Did I mention purple? I love purple. And I thought – a wee test drive wouldn't do any harm. And I just thought: 'Fuck it – I am having it. 9K more than I can afford but Fuck it. I WANT IT. And I got it. And I love it. My colleague, Jane, calls it a clit extension as opposed to the male equivalent of a dick extension. But do I give a shit? No – I LOVE IT.

Then I was on a roll. I always wanted bright red toenails and fingernails but never got them. And I suddenly remembered my lovely Granny saying women with red nails were whores. Has that stuck in my mind? But she also said that I'd go deaf if I had a bath when had my period. And that wasn't true. So Fuck It! An hour later I was driving my purple sports car with lovely red talons.

Tattoo is next on the list. Ten years ago I collapsed as my guts burst through my chest wall – it was like something from Alien. I was in Barcelona and rushed into emergency theatre to have my chest ripped open and everything crammed back in and stitched back up. I have little memory apart from the surgeon saying to my friend 'if we do not operate now she will not last more than a few hours'. I have a massive scar as a result. I am not ashamed of it – it is part of me and without it I would not be here and it reminds me of the kindness of family and friends (and strangers – will never forget the loveliest Spanish girl who put herself out to translate, sort insurance, sort flights, visit me, reassure me and so much more when she had only met me a few hours before). It also reminds me of experiencing vulnerability for the first time. I like bluebells and bumblebees lots – so am playing around with a design – the scar will be the stalk of the bluebell. Someone told me I need to think about what it will look like when I am 80. If I get to 80 I won't give a fuck what it looks like tbh. And I doubt anyone else will give a shit either.

My Fuck it list is growing – I want to sleep outside one night under the stars. I want to go up Carlton Hill at sunrise and have Bucks Fizz as I watch the sun come up. I want to go to Iona and out to Fingal's Cave. I want to sit on the beach at midnight with a Glayva and ice and listen to the waves. I want to have a go on the back of a motorbike along a coastal road (almost sorted that one – just getting a helmet coz I'm just practicing being wild at the moment and one must be a little sensible) It is a continually developing list – it will be updated, rejuvenated – a bit like myself.

Kim Cattrall says the menopause is the start of the next fabulous phase of our lives. I mean 'fabulous' might be a bit much – but I get the general concept. You are not too old and it's not too late.

So let's raise a glass to the women who never made it this far and let's do one Fuck It thing just for them.

Because if they could give advice they would tell you to have as many Fuck it moments as you possibly can.

43263826R00116

Printed in Poland
by Amazon Fulfillment
Poland Sp. z o.o., Wrocław